50 LANDMARK PAPERS

every
Oral & Maxillofacial Surgeon Should Know

50 LANDMARK PAPERS

every

Oral & Maxillofacial Surgeon Should Know

EDITED BY

Niall MH McLeod FRCS (OMFS), FDS, MRCS

Consultant Oral & Maxillofacial Surgeon
The Royal London and Whipps Cross Hospitals
London, UK

Peter A Brennan MD, PhD, FRCS, FRCSI, FDS

Consultant Maxillofacial Surgeon
Professor of Surgery
Queen Alexandra Hospital
Portsmouth, UK

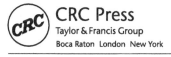

CRC Press
Taylor & Francis Group
Boca Raton London New York

CRC Press is an imprint of the
Taylor & Francis Group, an **informa** business

CRC Press
Boca Raton and London

First edition published 2020
by CRC Press
6000 Broken Sound Parkway NW, Suite 300, Boca Raton, FL 33487-2742

and by CRC Press
2 Park Square, Milton Park, Abingdon, Oxon, OX14 4RN

ISBN: 9780367254872 (hbk)
ISBN: 9780367210526 (pbk)
ISBN: 9780429288036 (ebk)

Typeset in Times New Roman MT Std
by KnowledgeWorks Global Ltd.

Contents

Section One   Anatomy

Section Two   Cancer

Section Three   Cleft

Section Four   Craniofacial

Section Five   Oral Medicine

Section Six   Oral Surgery

Section Seven   Orthognathic

Section Eight   Salivary

Section Nine   Skin

Section Ten   Temporomandibular Joint (TMJ)

Section Eleven   Trauma

Preface

The last 50 years has seen an exponential increase in the publication of research and new knowledge across medical and surgical disciplines. Our specialty of Oral and Maxillofacial Surgery (OMFS) continues to advance at a rapid pace, and with the number of information sources currently available, it can be difficult for both aspiring and established surgeons to know what is pertinent to their practice.

The "50 Landmark Papers in" series seeks to help busy clinicians by putting together a reference collection of well-respected papers and commentaries that could be considered important for the practice of a specialty. For trainees in particular, they provide a valuable resource prior to their specialty examination.

Choosing 50 papers that fulfil that brief has been extremely challenging, with such a broad range of subspecialty areas to choose from.

We decided not to follow such a rigid methodology as some books in this series, but instead asked 11 respected colleagues (listed below) to identify a series of papers that they thought were essential reading. Their choices were based on key developments in surgical practice, essential reviews of a topic, or the latest developments that are likely to be key for the future. These choices from colleagues produced an original list of 68 papers that we then reduced to 50 in an attempt to produce an even and balanced topic distribution covering the whole remit of OMFS.

There will not be a universal agreement on all of the papers that we have included in this book, but any debate this stimulates should be useful in identifying key papers that were missed for future editions.

As time passes, and surgical practice moves forward, these papers should remain useful historical references, and we hope that this book will, therefore, be a valuable resource for many years to come.

Niall MH McLeod
Peter A Brennan

List of colleagues who selected the essential reading list in the different subspecialties of OMFS

Anatomy
Madan Ethunandan
Consultant Oral & Maxillofacial Surgeon
Honorary Senior Clinical Lecturer
University Hospital Southampton
Southampton, UK

Cancer and Reconstruction
Anastasios Kanatas
Professor/Consultant Oral and Maxillofacial Surgeon
Leeds Teaching Hospitals
Leeds, UK

Cleft Lip and Palate
Simon van Eeden
Consultant Cleft and Oral and Maxillofacial Surgeon
Alder Hey Children's Hospital
and
Aintree University Hospital
Liverpool, UK

Craniofacial
David Richardson
Consultant Oral and Maxillofacial Surgeon
Maxillofacial Unit
Aintree University Hospital Craniofacial Unit
and
Alder Hey Children's Hospital
Liverpool, UK

Oral Medicine
Darryl Coombes
Consultant Maxillofacial Surgeon
The Nuffield Hospital
Tunbridge Wells, UK

Oral Surgery
Vinod Patel
Consultant Oral Surgeon
Guy's and St Thomas' Dental Institute
London, UK

Orthognathic
Greg J Knepil
Consultant Oral & Maxillofacial Surgeon
Gloucestershire Royal Hospital
Gloucester, UK

Salivary
Katherine S George
Consultant Oral & Maxillofacial Surgeon
King's College Hospital
London, UK

Skin Cancer
Darryl Godden
Consultant Oral & Maxillofacial Surgeon
Gloucestershire Royal Hospital
Gloucester, UK

Temporomandibular Joint Surgery
Nadeem R Saeed
Consultant Oral and Maxillofacial Surgeon
Great Ormond Street Hospital
London, UK
and
Oxford University Hospitals
Oxford, UK

Trauma
Simon Holmes
Consultant Oral & Maxillofacial Surgeon
Professor of Craniomaxillofacial Traumatology
The Royal London Hospital
London, UK

Contributors

Peyman Alam
Western Sussex Hospitals NHS
Foundation Trust
St Richards Hospital
Chichester, UK

Indran Balasundaram
London Northwest University NHS Trust
Imperial College NHS Trust
and
Hillingdon Hospital NHS Trust
Uxbridge, UK

Victoria Beale
Royal Manchester Children's Hospital
Manchester, UK

Raghuram Boyapati
Queen Victoria Hospital
East Grinstead, UK

Johno Breeze
University Hospitals Birmingham
Birmingham, UK

Peter A Brennan
Queen Alexandra Hospital
Portsmouth, UK

Alice Cameron
Royal United Hospitals Bath NHS
Foundation Trust
Bath, UK

Soudeh Chegini
London Deanery OMFS
London, UK

Alistair RM Cobb
University Hospitals Bristol NHS
Foundation Trust
Bristol, UK

Serryth Colbert
Royal United Hospitals Bath NHS
Foundation Trust
Bath, UK

Jag Dhanda
Queen Victoria Hospital
Imperial College London
Brighton and Sussex Medical School
East Grinstead, UK

Eric J Dierks
The Head and Neck Institute
Head and Neck Surgical Associates
Portland, Oregon

Stergios Doumas
Brighton and Sussex University
Hospitals NHS Trust
Brighton, UK

Jacob D'Souza
Royal Surrey County Hospital
Guildford, UK

Leander Dubois
Amsterdam UMC
Amsterdam, Netherlands

Harald Essig
Interdisciplinären Craniofazialen
Centrums der Universität Zürich (ICFC)
Zürich, Switzerland

Madan Ethunandan
University Hospital Southampton
Southampton, UK

Kathleen Fan
King's College Hospital
London, UK

Adrian Franke
University Hospital "Carl-Gustav Carus"
Technical University Dresden
Dresden, Germany

Cristina Frezzini
Sheffield Teaching Hospitals
NHS Foundation Trust
Sheffield, UK

Katherine S George
King's College Hospital
NHS Foundation Trust
London, UK

Ghaly A Ghaly
Dundee University
Ninewells Hospital
Dundee, Scotland

Peter T Glen
Gloucester Royal Hospital
Gloucester, UK

Daryl Godden
Gloucester Royal Hospital
Gloucester, UK

Siddharth Gowrishankar
The John Radcliffe Hospital
Oxford, UK

Lisa Greaney
Chelsea and Westminster and West
   Middlesex University Hospital
NHS Foundation Trust
London, UK

Jason Green
University Hospitals Birmingham
Birmingham, UK

David Grimes
Queen's Medical Centre
Nottingham, UK

Elizabeth A Gruber
Princess Alexandra Hospital
Harlow, UK

Emma Hayes
Kings's College Hospital
London, UK

Anusha Hennedige
Royal Manchester Children's Hospital
Manchester, UK

Cameron M Herbert
Guy's and St Thomas' NHS Foundation
   Trust
London, UK

Michael WS Ho
Leeds Teaching Hospitals NHS Trust
Leeds Dental Institute
Leeds, UK

Simon Holmes
Barts and the Royal London Hospitals
London, UK

Esther A Hullah
Faculty of Dentistry, Oral and
   Craniofacial Sciences
King's College
and
Guy's and St Thomas' NHS Foundation
   Trust
London, UK

Robert Isaac
Queen Alexandra Hospital
Portsmouth, UK

Anastasios Kanatas
Leeds Teaching Hospitals NHS Trust
and
St James's Institute of Oncology
Leeds, UK

Greg J Knepil
Gloucestershire Hospitals NHS
   Foundation Trust
Gloucestershire, UK

Jan de Lange
Amsterdam UMC/ACTA
University of Amsterdam
Amsterdam, Netherlands

Günter Lauer
University Hospital
Technische Universität Dresden
Dresden, Germany

Henry Leonhardt
University Hospital "Carl-Gustav Carus"
Technical University Dresden
Dresden, Germany

Derek Lowe
Evidence-Based Practice Research
  Centre (EPRC)
Edge Hill University
Ormskirk, UK
University Hospital Aintree
Liverpool, UK

Konstantinos Mantsopoulos
University of Erlangen-Nuremberg
Erlangen, Germany

David M McGoldrick
University Hospitals Birmingham NHS
  Foundation Trust
Birmingham, UK

Mark McGurk
University College Hospitals
London, UK

Alasdair McKechnie
University of Leeds
Leeds, UK

Kevin McMillan
RCDM Birmingham
Birmingham, UK

David A Mitchell
University of York
York, UK

Oliver Mitchell
Queen Alexandra Hospital
Portsmouth, UK

Florencio Monje
Medical School
Extremadura University
Badajoz, Spain

Rafal Niziol
King's College Hospital
London, UK

Graham R Oliver
Gloucesterhsire Hospitals
NHS Foundation Trust
Gloucesterhsire, UK

Neil J Opie
Chesterfield Royal Hospital NHS
  Foundation Trust
Derbyshire, UK

Vinod Patel
Guys Dental Hospital
London, UK

Mike Perry
Northwick Park Hospital
Harrow, UK

Toby Pitts-Tucker
Queen Alexandra Hospital
Portsmouth, UK

Pieter G Raijmakers
Amsterdam UMC
Amsterdam, Netherlands

Costa Repanos
Queen Alexandra Hospital
Portsmouth, UK

Ben Robertson
Liverpool University Dental Hospital
Liverpool, UK

Simon Rogers
Evidence-Based Practice Research
  Centre (EPRC)
Edge Hill University
Ormskirk, UK
and
University Hospital Aintree
Liverpool, UK

John Rowson
Nottingham University Hospitals
Nottingham, UK

Nadeem R Saeed
Great Ormond Street Hospital
London, UK
and
Oxford University Hospitals
Oxford, UK

Carrol P Saridin
HagaZiekenhuis
The Hague, Netherlands

Andrew Schache
University of Liverpool Cancer
   Research Centre
Liverpool, UK

Ruud Schreurs
Amsterdam UMC
Amsterdam, Netherlands

Andrew Sidebottom
Nottingham University
Nottingham, UK

Alistair G Smyth
Leeds Teaching Hospitals NHS Trust
Liverpool, UK

Tomas Svoboda
Queen Alexandra Hospital
Portsmouth, UK

Sundeep Thusu
London Deanery
London, UK

Simon van Eeden
Alder Hey Children's Hospital
Liverpool, UK

Baucke van Minnen
University Medical Center Groningen
Groningen, Netherlands

Jennifer Vesey
Liverpool University Dental Hospital
Liverpool, UK

Tom WM Walker
University Hospitals Bristol NHS
   Foundation Trust
Bristol, UK

Stephen Walsh
Western Sussex Hospitals NHS
   Foundation Trust
St Richards Hospital
Chichester, UK

Tatiana Welsch
Chelsea and Westminster and West
   Middlesex University Hospital
NHS Foundation Trust
London, UK

Surgical Anatomy of the Mandibular Ramus of the Facial Nerve Based on the Dissection of 100 Facial Halves

Dingman RO, Grabb WC. Plast Reconstr Surg. 1962; 29: 266–72.

Reviewed by Siddharth Gowrishankar

Research Question/Objective

To define the relations of the mandibular ramus (branch) of the facial nerve to the mandible to aid the surgeon in planning approaches to the body and ramus of the mandible.

Study Design

Anatomical study based on the dissection of 100 facial halves. Detailed drawings were made at the time of each dissection of the mandibular ramus and its relation to adjacent structures.

Sample Size

One-hundred facial halves.

Inclusion/Exclusion Criteria

The original article does not specify any information regarding specific inclusion or exclusion criteria.

Intervention or Treatment Received

One-hundred facial halves were dissected. Drawings were made at the time of dissection of the mandibular ramus and its relation to adjacent structures. Description of the mandibular ramus of the facial nerve presented under four headings:

    a. Its relationship with inferior border of the mandible
    b. Its relationship with posterior facial vein, anterior facial vein, and anterior facial artery
    c. The number of branches
    d. Its peripheral anastomosis with the buccal branch of the facial nerve

Results

The relationship of the mandibular ramus of the facial nerve with the inferior border of the mandible is conveniently divided into its course posterior and anterior to the facial artery.

Posterior to the facial artery, the mandibular ramus was seen to pass above the inferior border of the mandible in 81% of cases and in the 19% of cases that it passed below; its lowest point was within 1 cm of the inferior border.

Anterior to the facial artery, 100% of the branches which innervate the depressor muscles were above the lower the border of the mandible.

In 98% of the specimens, the nerve passed on the superficial surface of the posterior facial vein and in 2% deep to it.

One-hundred percent of the nerve passed superficial to the anterior facial vein.

Although most anatomy textbooks refer to the mandibular ramus of the facial nerve as a single nerve, this is true only in 21% of the cases. There were 2 major branches in 67% of cases, 3 major branches in 9%, and 4 major branches in 3% of cases. When there was more than one branch, the lowest nerve tended to be of the largest caliber.

Cross-innervation with the buccal branch of the facial nerve was seen in only 5% of cases.

Application, Significance and Usage

This was one of the earliest and seminal works which looked specifically at the anatomy of the mandibular ramus of the facial nerve in relation to surgical approaches to the body of the mandible.

Modern maxillofacial surgical practice encounters the mandibular branch of the facial nerve in numerous instances from limited exposure for open reduction of mandibular fractures through to wide exposure for neck dissections.

Of the five major peripheral branches of the facial nerve, the mandibular branch is the most frequently damaged in operations, due to a proportionally greater number of operations involving that region and the lack of anastomotic links with other branches.

Based on their study, the authors recommended skin incisions to approach the body of the mandible extra orally be placed at least one finger breadth or 2 cm below the lower border, along skin lines, to avoid damage to the mandibular ramus of the facial nerve.

In considering open reduction and internal fixation of the mandibular condyle, injury to the marginal mandibular branch of the facial nerve is a commonly cited complication. A recent meta-analysis reported the transmasseteric antero-parotid approach with retromandibular and preauricular extensions for condylar "neck" fractures was the safest in terms of facial nerve injury.[1,2]

Study Limitations

No specific information is provided regarding inclusion and exclusion criteria, age or sex of the dissected specimen, or the preservation or fixation techniques which can all affect the results.

No specific information regarding who performed the dissection, how the measurements were made, whether magnification was used during dissection or measurement, whether the mouths were opened or closed, whether there were any mandibular anomalies and dental status of the cadaver were given. There was also no information regarding whether the data was validated by repeat measurements by another observer.

No specific information is given regarding depth of the nerve and its relationship to the deep fascia of the neck.

Study and findings are based on two-dimensional anatomic dissection of preserved facial specimens and not physiologic in vivo measurements in a living person.

Relevant Studies

Earlier studies describing the anatomy of the facial nerve include ones published by Davis et al.[3] and Byars et al.[4] but they primarily described the course of the nerve in relation to the parotid gland.

Ziarah and Atkinson[5] in 1981 dissected 110 facial halves to look at the anatomy of the mandibular as well as cervical branch of the facial nerve.

There was reasonable congruence between their study and the Dingman and Grabb study with regard to the percentage of multiple nerve branches and also the relationship of the nerve with anterior facial vein (nerve always lies superficial to it).

Their findings however differed from the Dingman and Grabb study in the following significant ways:

Posterior to the facial artery, the mandibular ramus of the facial nerve was seen to pass above the inferior border of the mandible in 47% of cases only (compared to 81% of Dingman study), and in 53% of cases it passed below the mandible (lying as far below as 1.2 cm in one case).

Anterior to the facial artery, 6% of the nerves continued to run below the mandible (0% in the Dingman and Grabb study) for a distance of up to 1.5 cm (range of 0.8–1.5 cm) or as far forward as the second premolar. The lower pole of the parotid lay at a maximum distance of 1.8 cm behind and below the gonion. Incisions made 2 cm clear of the gonion will preserve the parotid pole and its contained nerves.

In addition they published on the depth of the nerve. They concluded that the cervical and mandibular branches run in a plane just deep to platysma but just superficial to the investing layer of deep cervical fascia.

They proposed the concept of a "danger zone" where the mandibular nerve is most likely to be injured. This is an area bound by a posterior line 2 cm behind the gonion, an anterior line up to the second premolar tooth, and an inferior line 2 cm below the mandible. For the cervical branch of the facial nerve, the anterior and posterior boundaries are identical but the inferior line is oblique (3 cm below the gonion and 4 cm below the mandibular antegonial notch).

Continuity of anterior fibres of platysma and the quadratus labii inferioris makes it feasible that they can contract as one unit and could explain the "pseudo-paralysis" of the lower lip which can occur with damage to the cervical branch of the facial nerve even when then mandibular ramus is undamaged. This too can profoundly affect smile as pointed out by Ellenbogen.[6]

Other recent studies on the mandibular branch of the facial nerve include Potgieter et al.,[7] Saylam et al.,[8] Kim et al.,[9] and Hazani et al.[10] (See Table 1.1.)

In 2016, Davies et al.[11] published a systematic literature review of the anatomical landmarks for localisation of the branches of the facial nerve. Their study included 320 articles of which 17 met the chosen criteria. Their conclusions were that there were many different methods presented to identify the course of the facial nerve, bony landmarks in general are more reliable, but further work is needed for accurate localisation of this complex nerve with many anatomic variations.

Table 1.1   Mandibular branch localisation in the literature

Author	Landmark Used	Measurement
Potgieter et al. (2005)	Angle of mandible and facial artery	Average distance 2.3 mm superior to angle of mandible
Saylam et al. (2007)	Anterior border of parotid, lobule of ear Angle of mandible	Nerve at anterior border of parotid at the level of mandibular angle or within 6 mm superior to the angle
Hazani et al. (2011)	Masseteric tuberosity	Nerve crossed the mandible at a mean distance of 3 cm anterior to masseteric tuberosity

Conclusion

Although the classic extra-oral approach to the mandible continues to recommend making the skin incision and superficial dissection 2 cm below the inferior border of the mandible to preserve the mandibular branch of the facial nerve as originally described by Dingman and Grabb, this is no longer applied as dogmatically and a number of approaches, particularly to the ramus of the mandible, advocate a higher dissection with a view to either identifying the branch and protecting it, or aiming just above it and retracting it down.

REFERENCES

1. Wilson AW, Ethunandan M, Brennan PA. Transmasseteric antero-parotid approach for open reduction and internal fixation of condylar fractures. Br J Oral Maxillofac Surg. 2005; 43: 57–60.
2. Al-Moraissi EA, Louvrier A, Colletti G, et al. Does the surgical approach for treating condylar fractures affect the rate of seventh cranial nerve injuries? A systematic review and meta-analysis based on a new classification for surgical approaches. J Craniomaxillofac Surg. 2018; 46: 398–412.
3. Davis RA, Anson BJ, Budinger JM, Kurth LE. Surgical anatomy of the facial nerve and parotid gland based upon a study of 350 cervicofacial halves. Surg Gynec Obs. 1956; 102: 385.
4. Byars LT. Preservation of the facial nerve in operations for benign conditions of the parotid area. Ann Surg. 1952; 136: 412–9.
5. Ziarah HÁ, Atkinson ME. The surgical anatomy of the cervical distribution of the facial nerve. Br J Oral Surg. 1981; 19: 171–9.
6. Ellenbogen R. Pseudo-paralysis of the mandibular branch of the facial nerve after platysmal face lift operation. Plast Reconstr Surg. 1979; 63: 364–8.
7. Potgieter W, Meiring JH, Boon JM, et al. Mandibular landmarks as an aid in minimizing injury to the marginal mandibular branch: a metric and geometric anatomical study. Clin Anat. 2005; 18: 71–8.
8. Saylam C, Ucerler H, Orhan M, Uckan A, Ozek C. Localization of the marginal mandibular branch of the facial nerve. J Craniofac Surg. 2007; 18: 137–42.
9. Kim DI, Nam SH, Nam YS, et al. The marginal mandibular branch of the facial nerve in Koreans. Clin Anat. 2009; 22: 207–14.
10. Hazani R, Chowdhry S, Mowlavi A, Wilhelmi BJ. Bony anatomic landmarks to avoid injury to the marginal mandibular nerve. Aesthet Surg J. 2011; 31: 286–9.
11. Davies JC, Agur AMR, Fattah AY. Anatomic landmarks for localisation of the branches of the facial nerve. OA Anatomy. 2013; 1: 33.

CHAPTER 2

The Superficial Musculo-Aponeurotic System (SMAS) in the Parotid and Cheek Area

Mitz V, Peyronie M. Plast Reconstr Surg. 1976; 58: 80–8.

Reviewed by Sundeep Thusu

Research Question/Objective

The "superficial muscular and aponeurotic system (SMAS)" is a fascial layer in the parotid and cheek regions which is described in classic anatomy textbooks such as Gray's[1] textbook of anatomy. In this paper, both the anatomical and potential surgical applications of the SMAS are considered.

Study Design

Fifteen fresh cadavers in total were studied. Of those seven were dissected into 14 hemifacial preparations. Additionally, three heads were serially sectioned into one of three planes – sagittal, frontal and horizontal. Each section was 1 cm thick with preparation to opacify the very small arteries and veins. Each section was then studied radiologically.

Another three heads were similarly sectioned without preparation and x-rayed.

Sample Size

Fifteen fresh cadavers.

Inclusion/Exclusion Criteria

All cadavers were over the age of 50.

Results

Facial dissection shows that the SMAS is stretched both superiorly and inferiorly. The SMAS is kept tensed superiorly by the superficial temporal muscles, the external part of the frontalis muscle, and the orbicularis oculi muscles. It is tensed inferiorly by the platysma muscle and attached posteriorly to the tragus and the mastoid area. Such a peripheral stretching explains how the SMAS could be an amplifier for the contractions of the facial muscles; the more it is tensed the less energy is required for the muscle to transmit contractions.

Furthermore, the SMAS transmits the actions of the facial muscles through two directions by acting as a distributor of all facial muscular contraction to the skin. Each muscle contraction follows one preferential direction in the network. An infinite number of resultant actions are possible because:

1. The SMAS relays the contractions of facial muscles along the longitudinal network parallel to the facial plane and
2. The SMAS transmits the resultant effect in a perpendicular direction towards the facial skin, through the fibrous expansions from the SMAS to the dermis.

Hence, the human face has the ability to express so many different nuances and shades of expression. Each expression of the facial is the result of several muscles, transmitted in combinations by the SMAS network to the skin.

Ageing weakens the elastic fibres of the SMAS and lessens the efficiency of the transmission of muscle contractions to the skin.

Macroscopic and Microscopic Structure of SMAS

The SMAS can be divided into two broad areas: the parotid area and the cheek area.

In the parotid area the SMAS is a condensed mesh, distinct from the fascia of the parotid gland. Adherent to the pre-tragal area for 1 or 2 cm the SMAS then becomes separate from the parotid sheath.

Microscopically the SMAS is composed of one to three layers between the parotid fascia proper and the skin. Sometimes the muscular fibres are obvious within the fibrous layer hence the term muscular-aponeurotic system.

In the cheek area, the SMAS becomes thinner and can be only be followed macroscopically. Underneath the dermis, the SMAS is a continuous fibrous net sending several extensions out to the dermis. This network constantly covers the facial muscles. Hence, the SMAS comprises all the attachments from these muscles to the dermis.

Relationship of the SMS to the Other Facial Structures

Nerves In the parotid area, only sensory nerves (branches of the anterior cervical plexus) are located within the dermis and the SMAS. The facial nerve and its branches run deep into the parotid glands and are protected by the parotid fascia and the external lobe of the gland.

In the cheek area, the facial motor nerves run deeper than the SMAS and the only nerves that go through the SMAS are sensory nerves. Motor branches reach the superficial layer of the facial muscles through their deeper aspect.

An important layer of fat is often located between the SMAS and the dermis, which is completely separated from Bichat's fat pad by the SMAS.

Muscles The SMAS invests and extends into the external part of the superficial facial muscles, involving fibres of the risorius, the frontalis, the platysma and the peripheral part of the orbicularis oculi.

Vessels The facial artery and vein lie deep to the SMAS with their perforating branches go through it and the subdermal vascular network lies superficial to it. Hence the SMAS forms the deep border of the neurovascular and muscular cutaneous complex.

The Parotid Glands In the pre-tragal area, the SMAS and the parotid fibrous fascia are united in a dense layer of connective tissue. Here a surgical dissection of the SMAS is possible and safe. Anteriorly, the SMAS is completely independent of the fibrous fascia surrounding the parotid gland. However, because it is thin and covers the motor nerve branches, the surgical dissection anteriorly is difficult and dangerous.

Zygomatic Area The SMAS crosses in front of the zygomatic arch and belongs to the temporozygomatic SMAS, which adheres to the periosteum. The superior frontal branch of the facial nerve lies deep to SMAS; the sensory nerve branches run between the SMAS and the dermis. The space overlying the external part of the zygomatic arch is very narrow, so dissection of the SMAS is both difficult and dangerous.

Mandibular Area Here the SMAS is in close contact with the superficial fibres of platysma. A safe plane of dissection is found deep to the platysma and the SMAS as the mandibular branch of the facial nerve runs deeper here.

Mastoid Area The SMAS is intimately attached to the dermis and to the fibrous tissue around the inserts of the sternoclavicular muscles. It is rather difficult to isolate the SMAS around the ear because the various fibrous layers are closely entwined.

Surgical Applications of the SMAS
Preventing Facial Palsy Experience with cadaver dissection showed that careful consideration must be taken to avoid damage to the branches of the facial nerve. It was found that injuries to the facial nerve commonly occurred during a retrofascial dissection where either the SMAS layer is thin, or the superficial lobe of the parotid is short and does not protect the nerves, or whereby the dissection is carried out too far forward (beyond the anterior border of the parotid glands).

To avoid facial paralysis from injury to the facial nerve, dissection should be in front of the tragus and dissecting scissors inserted between the SMAS and the parotid fascia. The SMAS is carefully freed from this fascia which becomes easy once the proper plane is found.

Dissection should not be carried further upward than 1 cm below the zygomatic arch or lower than 1 cm above the inferior margin of the mandible. Once the SMAS is freed from the parotid fascia, it becomes possible to lift the face much more easily and safely.

Face-Lift Cadaveric dissection found that the SMAS in the pre-tragal region is in continuity with the lateral end of the frontalis muscle in the upper part of the face and with the platysma muscle in the lower face and neck. Fibrous septa extending from the SMAS to the dermis through the subcutaneous fat create a wide mesh of connections between the skin of the cheek and the underlying SMAS. The surgical undermining at the superficial subcutaneous plane as is done in the classic face-lift procedure destroys these fibrous connections between the SMAS and skin. Consequently, the laxity of the deeper tissues that sag with the skin is not corrected by rhytidoplasty alone.

While the SMAS and platysma are interconnected with the skin and subcutaneous tissue, the under surface of this anatomic flap is not intimately fixed to the deeper structures. A potentially avascular space is present between the superficial flap and the external layer of the deep cervical fascia of the neck, which continues into the cheek as the true parotid fascia. Due to this anatomic configuration, the SMAS-platysma layer is easily separated from the deep cervical fascia. Almost no vessels cross this plane. This deeper fascial dissection respects the function of the SMAS and it allows a stronger pullback of the fascia and skin together. When the excess part of the SMAS is resected and sutured to the pre-tragal area, the anterior muscles and the skin may be pulled back (or "lifted"). This approach also lessens the area which has to be undermined, as only the parotid area has to be freed to obtain this pullback.

Study Limitations

Similar studies today would have made use of other modalities of imaging such as CT or MRI to aid in soft tissue anatomy.

Relevant Studies

Incorporating the anatomic descriptions of this paper with the surgical technique of sub-platysmal dissection originally advocated in classical face-lifts,[2] Owsley devised the technique of SMAS-platysma face-lift in which the redundant tissue of the cheek, jaw-line and neck are lifted by freeing the upwards advancement of the compound flap comprising the interconnected skin and SMAS-platysma layer.[3-5]

Extensive experience with this technique has shown several advantages of the SMAS-platysma face-lift operation with temporary injury of the facial nerve. Analysis of 322 consecutive cases of platysma-SMAS face-lift over a 4-year period indicated that nine patients had a temporary decrease in function of the platysma muscle, characterised by diminished depressor activity of the chin.[5] This was related to dysfunction of either the cervical branch of the facial nerve or the platysma muscle due to transection.[6] The temporary deformity was minimal, and the patients recovered full function within 3 months. There were no instances of injury to the marginal mandibular, buccal or frontal branches of the facial nerve. The frequency of nerve injury with the SMAS-platysma operation is comparable to that published in other series in which the classical face-lift procedure was done.[7]

Knowledge of the mid facial ligaments provided an improved understanding of the support system of the facial soft tissues and the role they played in the ageing process.[8]

More modifications of the face-lift ensued culminating in a focus on retaining ligament release in a sub SMAS, or deep plane dissection as well as developing subperiosteal techniques for facial soft tissue repositioning with the primary goal of re-suspending descended malar fat to the malar eminence.[9–11]

REFERENCES

1. Gray H. Anatomy of the Human Body, 25th ed. Philadelphia, PA: Lea & Febiger, 1949.
2. Skoog T. Plastic Surgery – New Methods and Refinements. Philadelphia, PA: WB Saunders Co, 1974.
3. Owsley JQ Jr. Platysma-fascial rhytidectomy. Plast Reconstr Surg. 1977; 60: 843–50.
4. Owsley JQ Jr. Platysma-SMAS rhytidectomy, a four year experience. In Gradihger G, Kaye B (Eds): Symposium on Problems and Complications in Aesthetic Plastic Surgery of the Face. St. Louis: CV Mosby Co., 1984.
5. Owsley JQ Jr. Discussion of Souther SG, Vistnes LM: Medial approximation of the platysma muscle in the treatment of neck deformities. Plast Reconstr Surg. 1981; 67: 614–5.
6. Ellenbogen R. Pseudo-paralysis of the mandibular branch of the facial nerve after platysmal face-lift operation. Plast Reconstr Surg. 1979; 63: 364–8.
7. Baker DC, Conley J. Avoiding facial nerve injuries in rhytidectomy-anatomical variations and pitfalls. Plast Reconstr Surg. 1979; 64: 781–95.
8. Furnas DW. The retaining ligaments of the cheek. Plast Reconstr Surg. 1989; 83: 11–6.
9. Tessier P. Face-lifting and frontal rhytidectomy. In Ely JF (Ed.): Transactions of the Seventh International Congress of Plastic and Reconstructive Surgery. Rio de Janeiro, 1980.

10. Psillakis JM, Rumley TO, Camargos A. Subperiosteal approach as an improved concept for correction of the aging face. Plast Reconstr Surg. 1988; 82: 383–94.
11. Ramirez OM, Maillard GF, Musolas A. The extended subperiosteal face lift: a definitive soft-tissue remodeling for facial rejuvenation. Plast Reconstr Surg. 1991; 88: 227–36. discussion 237–38.

CHAPTER 3

Post-Traumatic Orbital Reconstruction: Anatomical Landmarks and the Concept of the Deep Orbit

Evans BT, Webb AA. Br J Oral Surg. 2007; 45: 183–9.

Reviewed by Simon Holmes

Research Question/Objective

This paper aims to demystify the surgical approaches to the orbit, and to objectify safe surgical procedures to enable full dissection and exposure of the fracture configuration with minimal risk to important anatomical structures.

Study Design

This is an opinion paper following a review of literature and considerable surgical experience.

Sample Size

Not applicable.

Follow-up

Not applicable.

Inclusion/Exclusion Criteria

Not applicable.

Intervention or Treatment Received

Not applicable.

Results

The management of orbital trauma has evolved considerably in the last decade. Advances in diagnosis have followed considerable improvements in imaging to enable precise and detailed knowledge of orbital fracture patterns.

The concept of orbital volume and recognition of its importance has been helpful to conceptualise management; in addition, increasing awareness of the important three-dimensional shape of the floor and medial wall to maintain globe projection has driven reconstructive techniques.[1]

With advances in surgical access[2,3] and landmark papers in orbital bone analysis[4] leading to preformed anatomical plates,[5] the surgeon now has an armamentarium potentially able to replicate three-dimensional anatomy with a degree of perfection.

This paper attempts to guide the surgeon along a safe surgical path to achieve the anatomical ideal. The senior author was an incredibly experienced orbital surgeon and keen anatomist. This interest aroused observations of applied surgical anatomy of the orbit. Established orthodoxy led to the concept of safe distances, these being derived from dried adult skulls. The authors emphatically debunk these concepts, citing that in the trauma case particularly with loss of the orbital rim, or medial margin, not only is there no origin to measure from, but in addition the anatomical variation makes these measurements meaningless. In addition, I would cite that the anterior and posterior ethmoidal vessels emerge into the orbit at the junction of the ethmoid and frontal bone, and are therefore incredibly difficult to reach surgically. It should also be remembered that the vessels themselves if damaged are likely to be thrombosed in the time interval between injury and surgery.

It is therefore more useful to define anatomically the key areas for surgical isolation to achieve good reconstruction and then provide a way to expose them safely.

Following clarification of the importance of subperiosteal dissection, the paper describes the deep orbit as commencing at the origin of the inferior orbital fissure. This is readily identified surgically. Following exposure of this region, a reliable and robust second landmark is the infraorbital nerve, which is usually intact, and because this runs in a stereotypical direction, it is easily separated from the orbital periosteum, providing a means of predictable dissection.

As increased exposure is required, the authors identify the need to mobilise the orbital contents via division of the contents of the inferior orbital fissure. This is a crucial principle and allows increased surgical access, as well as aiding hemostasis.

In addition to the soft issue anatomy, the paper gives strong logical advice about facilitating subperiosteal dissection by the applied anatomy of the sphenoid bone. While the observation that the lateral wall of the orbit provides a very reliable means of checking reduction, the paper emphasises that the robust nature of the orbit at this point allows for a more reliable way to obtain a subperiosteal plane of dissection. It is indeed a truism that "the lateral wall is your friend" when starting out on the surgical apprenticeship and embarking on orbital reconstruction.

The applied surgical anatomy of the sphenoid bone is discussed and reference is made to the significance of a segmentation of the sphenoid bone with respect to injuries which are sight threatening. While this is not strictly covered by the title of the paper, it is extremely useful advice. The term sphenoid trigone is used, and in my view, it is extremely important to consider in high-energy transfers to signpost the risk of optic nerve neuropathy. This is physically helpful in counseling relatives in unconscious patients that there may well be significant morbidity.

The importance of the articulation of the zygomatic bone and sphenoid is recognised as one of the key areas to check reconstruction. On occasion this is technically challenging, and the paper goes on to discuss the benefits of a postero-lateral approach via a coronal flap and detachment of temporalis muscle. It is therefore possible to approach the lateral orbital floor from this aspect to facilitate safe dissection.

The posterior limit of the safe dissection rests with the orbital plate of the palatine bone, a relatively strong structure which provides a constant landmark and a convenient place to seat the posterior limit of the reconstruction material.

It is the posterior dissection which is potentially the most hazardous part of the procedure, and the paper recognises this.

On occasion, the footplate of the palatine bone can be small, and not readily identifiable, and in these circumstances the paper describes placing an instrument at the posterior wall of the maxillary sinus and tracing it superiorly until the palatine bone is encountered or to the level of the infraorbital nerve. Surgeons who cite the use of an endoscope to support their dissection could do well to consider this.[6]

Following dissection of these key areas, the floor of the orbit is considered fully exposed. The paper does not address exposure of the medial wall directly (see below), but it does go on to highlight the lack of constancy in position of the anterior and posterior ethmoidal vessels, which precludes their use in any meaningful way in surgical planning.

This paper is presented in a very readable format and is in my view a prerequisite for any trainee embarking on this surgery. If fully understood and enacted, surgical exposure can be conducted in a predictable and safe manner.

Study Limitations

Ultimately, the paper is limited because it is a personal interpretation following a significant and long-standing surgical career. This does not take away its importance in the literature, and it remains a keystone article on the subject.

While the paper does not address the medial wall approach, which weakens the article, it must be appreciated that at the time the article was written, this was an evolving area.[7] It is important to appreciate that medial wall exploration is conducted more efficiently and predictably following surgical exposure of the floor. Inevitably, it is important to consider navigation technology in the context of this article,[8] which was something that the senior author had a very strong view of, and considered that knowledge of anatomy, together with establishing strong landmarks, precluded routine use of this technology. I personally hold with this view – mostly – although it is very useful in larger reconstructions with margins in close proximity to the optic canal. This debate will resonate in scientific meetings for some time to come.

REFERENCES

1. Choi SH, Kang DH. Prediction of late enophthalmos using preoperative orbital volume and fracture area measurements in blowout fracture. J Craniofac Surg. 2017; 28: 1717–20.
2. Bähr W, Bagambisa FB, Schlegel G, Schilli W. Comparison of transcutaneous incisions used for exposure of the infraorbital rim and orbital floor: a retrospective study. Plast Reconstr Surg. 1992; 4: 585–91.
3. De Riu G, Meloni SM, Gobbi R, Soma D, Baj A, Tullio A. Subciliary versus swinging eyelid approach to the orbital floor. J Craniomaxillofac Surg. 2008; 36: 439–42.
4. Metzger MC, Schön R, Tetzlaf R, et al. Topographical CT-data analysis of the human orbital floor. Int J Oral Maxillofac Surg. 2007; 36: 45–53.
5. Scolozzi P, Momjian A, Heuberger J, et al. Accuracy and predictability in use of AO three-dimensionally preformed titanium mesh plates for posttraumatic orbital reconstruction: a pilot study. J Craniofac Surg. 2009; 20: 1108–13.
6. Park J, Huh J, Lee J, et al. Reconstruction of large orbital posterior floor wall fracture considering orbital floor slope using endoscope. J Craniofac Surg. 2017; 28: 947–50.
7. Choi M, Flores RL. Medial orbital wall fractures and the transcaruncular approach. J Craniofac Surg. 2012; 23: 696–701.
8. Markiewicz MR, Dierks EJ, Bell RB. Does intraoperative navigation restore orbital dimensions in traumatic and post-ablative defects? J Craniomaxillofac Surg. 2012; 40: 142–8.

CHAPTER 4

A Modified Pre-Auricular Approach to the Temporomandibular Joint and Malar Arch

Al-Kayat A, Bramley P. Br J Oral Surg. 1979; 17: 91–103.

Reviewed by Oliver Mitchell and Madan Ethunandan

Research Question/Objective

Analyse the position of the facial nerve in relation to easily identifiable landmarks. Improve the visibility and safety of the surgical approach to the zygomatic arch and temporomandibular joint (TMJ).

Study Design

Anatomical dissection of facial halves with observations recorded. All measurements were taken by one observer and the accuracy of observations checked against a second observer. These findings were then used to describe a new surgical approach to the zygomatic arch and TMJ.

Sample Size

56 facial halves (18 female, 10 male cadavers).

Intervention or Treatment Received

Anatomical dissection: The facial nerve trunk and its branches were dissected and its relationship to specific landmarks recorded. The anatomy of the temporal fascia was also assessed.

Landmarks chosen (Figure 4.1):

Point C: the most anterior concavity of the bony external auditory canal

Point Z: the point on the lateral surface of the zygomatic arch midway between its upper and lower border, where the most posterior branch of the temporal branch of the facial nerve crosses the arch

Point B: the lowest concavity of the bony external auditory canal

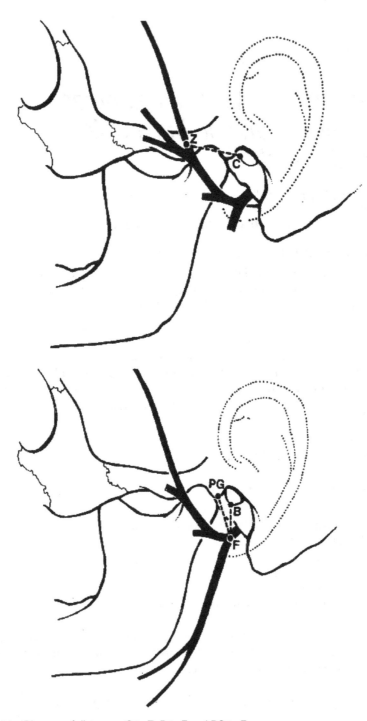

Figure 4.1   Diagram of distances C to Z, B to F and PG to F.

Point F: the point at which the facial nerve bifurcates into temporo-facial and cervico-facial divisions

Point PG: the lowest point of the post-glenoid tubercle

Results

Points	C to Z	B to F	PG to F
Number of observations	54	20	20
Mean	2.0 +/− 0.5 cm	2.3 +/− 0.28 cm	3.0 +/− 0.31 cm
Range	0.8–3.5 cm	1.5–2.8 cm	2.4–3.5 cm

Observations on the Temporal Fascia

- Superiorly the temporal fascia is a single, thick layer attached to the entire extent of the superior temporal line. At about 2 cm above the zygomatic arch the temporal fascia divides into two layers, one of which is attached to the lateral aspect of the periosteum of the zygomatic arch while the other is attached to the medial aspect.
- Contained between the two layers are a small quantity of fat, the zygomatic branch of the superficial temporal artery, and the zygomatico-temporal branch of the trigeminal nerve.
- At the level of the zygomatic arch, the periosteum firmly blends with both the outer layer of the temporal fascia and the superficial temporal fascia. This fusion of these three layers forms a tough connective tissue through which run the temporal and zygomatic branches of the facial nerve. In all cases it was difficult to dissect out the nerves without damaging them.
- As the temporal branch ascends in a supero-anterior direction, it becomes more superficial. It lies in the superficial fascia of the temporal region, together with the superficial temporal vessels and the auriculo-temporal nerve.

New Surgical Approach

- A "question mark" shaped incision was made in the temporal region with an inferior preauricular/end aural extension (Figure 4.2). The temporal component is made posterior to the temporal vessels and is carried through the skin and superficial temporal fascia to the level of the deep temporal fascia. Blunt dissection in this plane is carried downwards to a point about 2 cm above the zygomatic arch where the temporal fascia splits and contains fatty tissue, which is easily visible through the thin lateral layer. Beyond this point, there should be no attempt at further dissection of the superficial fascia from the temporal fascia. Starting at the root of the zygomatic arch, an incision running at 45° upwards and forwards is made through the superficial layer of the temporal fascia. Once inside this pocket, the periosteum

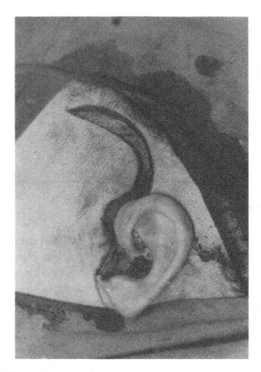

Figure 4.2   Skin incision.

of the zygomatic arch can be safely incised and turned forwards as one flap with the outer layer of temporal fascia and the superficial fascia. Proceeding downwards from the lower border of the arch and articular fossa, the tissues lateral to the joint capsule are dissected and retracted and the TMJ and the condyle can be exposed.

Study Limitations

Small number of cadavers dissected, and the suggested surgical technique was only used in five patients. Measurements at risk of observer bias.

Relevant Studies

Al-Kayat and Bramley's description of the anatomy of the temporal scalp, particularly the position of the most posterior branches of the temporal branches of the facial nerve, has provided a clear anatomical basis on which to develop surgical access to the TMJ.

The "perceived" complexity of the anatomy of the temporal scalp, especially the relationship of the layers of the temporal fascia to the periosteum overlying the zygomatic arch and to the position of the temporal branch of the facial nerve, has generated numerous surgical techniques to improve access and reduce morbidity. The described techniques could be scrutinised as those describing (a) improved access, (b) reduction in morbidity of the facial nerve, and (c) reduction in temporal hollowing.

Access

Many approaches to the TMJ have been described, but in their originally described format most fail to provide wide exposure of the TMJ and condylar area without excessive morbidity, with individual techniques having their own specific limitations and complications.[1]

The pre-auricular approach was popularised by Rowe, and Popowich and Crane described a technique with a limited temporal component, a vertical incision through the temporal fascia to the root of the zygomatic arch, but with similar planes of dissections as that described by Al-Kayat and Bramley.[2,3] Pogrel et al. described a bicoronal flap approach to the TMJ, which also provided wide exposure, but which requires a significantly wider dissection.[4]

Al-Kayat and Bramley's "?" incision, with a temporal component curving forward, provided wide exposure of the TMJ, with minimal cosmetic consequence as a significant proportion of the scar was hidden within the hairline.[1]

Reduction of Morbidity to the Facial Nerve

There was a high incidence of facial nerve injury reported in earlier descriptions of access the TMJ by House et al. (15%)[5], Dingman et al. (55%)[6], and Dolwick (32%).[7] Hall et al. compared supra-fascial and sub-fascial dissection techniques to access the TMJ and reported a reduction from 25% to 1.7% when a supra-fascial approach was changed to a sub-fascial approach.[8] Politi et al. described a "deep sub-fascial" approach to the TMJ, utilising a pre-auricular incision, with dissection between the deep temporal fascia and temporalis muscle and reported excellent aesthetic results with no injuries to the facial nerve.[9]

The relevance of the temporal scalp anatomy has also been highlighted by authors in evaluating the outcome of coronal flaps. The classical description of surgical techniques in the temporal region involves a plane of dissection between the superficial temporal (temporoparietal) fascia and the outer layer of the temporal fascia to minimise injury to the facial nerve. Gabrielli et al. reported a 11% incidence of facial nerve weakness following coronal flaps.[10] Kleinberger et al. evaluated a "deeper" plane of dissection between the undivided temporal fascia and the temporalis muscle when raising a coronal flap and highlighted the lack of facial nerve injury associated with this approach.[11]

The position of the facial nerve more anteriorly in the temporal region is of importance in facial cosmetic surgery, especially in the various face-lift-type procedures. In addition to the landmarks described by Al-Kayat and Bramley, the other authors have described the anatomy of the extracranial facial nerve in this area. Pitanguay's line describes the trajectory of the temporal branch on a line from 0.5 cm below the tragus to 1.5 cm above the lateral eyebrow.[12] Furnas describes the most posterior temporal branch crossing the superior border of the zygoma at a point 5 mm posterior to where a vertical projection of the anterior temporal hairline descends to the cross the zygoma.[13]

This landmark paper by Al-Kayat and Bramley has had a direct and indirect influence on surgical approaches to the craniofacial skeleton and TMJ. The evolution of any procedure is based on a sound anatomical basis and a critical evaluation of outcomes. Though it is less frequently used in its "originally" described format, its modifications and implications continue to play an important role in access to this area.

Postscript

There has and continues to be confusion in the terminology used to describe the various layers of the scalp in the temporal region. They are often and (sometimes) incorrectly used in an interchangeable manner. Following are the most frequent synonyms for terms utilised in this article.

> *Temporal fascia*—(Syn: Undivided temporal fascia, temporalis fascia, deep temporal fascia)
> *Outer layer of temporal fascia*—(Syn: Superficial layer of deep temporal fascia, superficial layer of temporal fascia)
> *Inner layer of temporal fascia*—(Syn: Deep layer of deep temporal fascia, deep layer of temporal fascia)
> *Superficial temporal fascia*—(Syn: Temporoparietal fascia, suprazygomatic SMAS)

REFERENCES

1. Al-Kayat A, Bramley P. A modified pre-auricular approach to the temporomandibular joint and malar arch. Br J Oral Surg. 1979; 17: 91–103.
2. Rowe NL. Surgery of the temporomandibular joint. Proc Roy Soc Med. 1972; 65: 383–8.
3. Popowich L, Crane RM. Modified preauricular access to the temporomandibular apparatus. Oral Surg Oral Med Oral Pathol. 1982; 54: 257–62.
4. Pogrel MA, Perrott DH, Kaban LB. Bicoronal flap approach to the temporomandibular joints. Int J Oral Maxillofac Surg. 1991; 20: 219–22.
5. House LR, Morgan DH, Hale WP. Clinical evaluation of TMJ arthroplasties with insertion of articular eminence prosthesis on ninety patients (an eight-year study). Laryngosocope. 1977; 87: 1182–7.

6. Dingman RO, Dingman DL, Lawrence RA. Surgical correction of lesions of the temporomandibular joints. Plast Reconstr Surg. 1975; 55: 335–40.

7. Dolwick MF, Kretzschmar DP. Morbidity associated with the preauricular and perimeatal approaches to the temporomandibular joint. J Oral Maxillofac Surg. 1982; 40: 699–700.

8. Hall MB, Brown RW, Lebowitz MS. Facial nerve injury during surgery of the temporomandibular joint: a comparison of two dissection techniques. J Oral Maxillofac Surg. 1985; 43: 20–3.

9. Politi M, Toro C, Cian R, Costa F, Robiny M. The deep subfascial approach to the temporomandibular joint. J Oral Maxillofac Surg. 2004; 62: 1097–102.

10. Gabrielli MP, Monnazzi MS, Gabrielli MF, et al. Clinical evaluation of the bicoronal flap in the treatment of facial fractures. Retrospective study of 132 patients. J Craniomaxillofac Surg. 2012; 40: 51–4.

11. Kleinberger AJ, Jumaily J, Speigel JH. Safety of modified coronal approach with dissection deep to temporalis fascia for facial nerve preservation. Otolaryngol Head Neck Surg. 2015; 152: 655–60.

12. Pitanguy I, Ramos AS. The frontal branch of the facial nerve: the importance of its variations in face lifting. Plast Reconstr Surg. 1966; 38: 352–6.

13. Furnas DW. Landmarks for the trunk and the temporofacial division of the facial nerve. Br J Surg. 1965; 52: 694–6.

CHAPTER 5

Bone Healing and Revascularisation after Total Maxillary Osteotomy

Bell WH, Fonseca RJ, Kenneky JW, Levy BM. J Oral Surg. 1975; 33: 253–60.

Reviewed by Ghaly A Ghaly

Research Question/Objective

This was an attempt to identify some of the problems and elucidate the process of wound healing after total maxillary osteotomy. The results of experiments in animals and clinical studies show that palatal mucosa and labial-buccal gingiva provide an adequate nutrient pedicle for single-stage total maxillary osteotomies.

Study Design

A total maxillary osteotomy was performed in adult male rhesus monkeys. The process included using an incision at the mucoperiosteal junction from one maxillary tuberosity to the other. A horizontal supra-nasal osteotomy was performed from the mediolateral aspect of the nasal aperture to the pterygomaxillary suture. Osteotomies were performed between nasal septum and superior surface of maxilla. The maxilla remained pedicled to the intact palatal mucosa and bucco-labial gingiva. An attempt was made to preserve the greater palatine artery in all but three of the animals, in which these vessels were intentionally transected during surgery. After mobilising the maxilla, the teeth were put on their preoperative occlusion without intermaxillary fixation. There is no mention of fixation of the mobilized maxilla. Wounds were closed with interrupted 3-0 silk sutures.

At animal sacrifice the carotid arteries were used in infuse Micropaque™ injection mediums in normal saline followed by Micropaque infusion in 10% formalin.

Sample Size

Twelve adult male resus monkeys. Seven had osteotomies with preservation of the greater palatine artery, three had transections of the greater palatine artery, and two were kept as controls.

Follow-up

The seven monkeys were killed at the following intervals; immediately, 2 days; and 1, 2, 4, 6 and 12 weeks after surgery. Of the three monkeys with the severed greater palatine artery, one was killed immediately, one at 4 weeks, and one at 6 weeks after surgery.

Inclusion/Exclusion Criteria

Male adult rhesus monkeys 8–14 years of age with average weight of 10.5 kg.

Intervention or Treatment Received

Total maxillary osteotomy, with or without preservation of the greater palatine artery.

Results

Postoperative course of all animals was uncomplicated, without signs of infection. Transient ischemia was noticed in the soft tissue incision edges and lasted for two to three days. The osteotomised maxillae stabilised within three weeks postoperatively. The individual teeth in the maxillae remained stable. In the animals euthanised immediately and at two days, the pulp of the inadvertently sectioned long canines was not perfused. The Micropaque infusant was present in the pulps of all the other teeth. Intraosseous circulatory embarrassment was noticed in nasomaxillary region and the bone encasing the canines. There was evidence that the recovery has started in the two days animal by a decrease in ischemia. In the one-week specimens there was increase in the filling of the endosteal and periosteal vascular beds. Specimens at two weeks showed the infusion medium to be well distributed in the bone and pulps of all maxillary teeth apart from the maxillary canines. The 4-week specimens showed distinct proliferation of the endosteal and periosteal circulatory beds. Despite the fact the apices of the maxillary canines were transected, the apical portion of the dental osseus segment remained viable and vascularised. The difference between the 4- and 6-week specimens were quantitative. The 12-week specimens showed vascular architecture comparable to the control specimens. Osseous bridging appeared to be complete by that stage. Bilateral ligation of the greater palatine arteries had no discernible effect on perfusion of Micropaque through the intrapulpal or soft tissues.

The study showed that blood supply for the maxilla during total osteotomy can be reliable via the buccal and palatal soft tissue flaps. In addition, it showed that ligation of the greater palatine artery had no effect on the survival of the maxilla. Evidence of bone healing is seen as early as six weeks after surgery.

Study Limitations

Performed on animals, not on humans. It also had a small sample size with one surgical technique. There was no consistency in numbers between the interventional groups and the controls. Some subjects in the group which did not have ligation of greater palatine artery were followed for a longer time.

The study also notes that as a practical matter the greater palatine artery might have been transected in all subjects intraoperatively.

Relevant Studies

Maxillary osteotomies were originally described in the 19th century for access to the nasopharynx, but it was not until the early 20th century that the Le Fort 1 osteotomy was first described for the correction of facial deformity by Wassmund.[1,2]

Due to concerns about the vascular supply of the maxilla, early techniques described a limited separation and mobilisation of the maxilla and were generally unstable. Many techniques used palatal incisions for access, which severely compromises the vascularity of the anterior maxilla, before Kole in 1959, amongst others, described a vestibular incision to improve access and protect the vascularity.[3] Later in 1965, Obwegeser described complete mobilisation of the maxilla and repositioning without tension using a wide vestibular incision, which has become the standard for maxillary osteotomy techniques.[4]

Bell, and Bell and Levy had already investigated revascularisation and bone healing in different single-stage anterior, posterior, and total maxillary osteotomy techniques using primates and the rhesus monkey was considered an excellent experimental model to develop new biologically sound maxillary surgical orthodontic techniques.[5-7]

Another study on the vascularity of anterior maxillary osteotomies by Nelson and coworkers found no significant difference between labial pedicle, tunnelling, and palatal pedicles.[8]

This study demonstrated evidence of the safety of the technique most commonly used for Le Fort 1 osteotomies and that buccal and palatal soft tissue flaps were adequate for the blood supply of the maxilla during this procedure. At the time, this study provided much-needed evidence for such procedures using animal models, The same process with modifications was subsequently used to prove healing after segmental maxillary osteotomy. This showed that the soft tissue flap provided adequate blood supply to the anterior maxillary segment when all bony segments were mobilised, with only transient effects on bone healing and viability.[9,10]

One criticism of such studies is that the maxillary segment(s) are not displaced during the surgery, and the effect of such displacement and stretching of the soft tissues on the vascularity of the maxilla is not clear. Recently the use of laser Doppler flowmetry permitted studies on patients showing that ligation of the descending palatine artery didn't influence maxillary gingival blood flow during Le Fort 1 osteotomy.[11]

Despite this, avascular necrosis of the maxilla remains a concern in orthognathic surgery, and a number of cases of partial or total necrosis are described in the literature.[12,13] Maxillary necrosis may arise due to excessive extension of the vestibular incision posteriorly, or disruption of the lesser palatine artery, the risk of which can be minimised by careful surgical technique.

There is a particular concern in patients with a cleft palate where the vascularity of the maxilla is compromised by the altered anatomy and by previous surgical procedures.[14]

•

Maxillary osteotomies using a tunneled technique had historically been described for segmental osteotomies, and have been proposed for osteotomies in cleft patients, but due to the limited visibility provided, they have are not routinely used in many centres.[2,15]

The vestibular access to the maxilla is of course also the principal approach for midfacial trauma, and the anatomical basis for the safety of this approach is demonstrated by this study.[16]

REFERENCE

1. Langenbeck B. Beitrange zur Osteoplastik – Die osteoplastiche resection der Oberkierers. Deutsche Klinik. In Goschen A (Hrsg) A, (Ed). Berlin: Reimer, 1859.
2. Wassmund M. Frakturen und Lurationen des Gesichtsschadels. Leipzig: Meusser Verlag, 1927.
3. Kole H. Surgical operations on the alveolar ridge to correct occlusal abnormalities. Oral Surg. Oral Surg Oral Med Oral Path. 1959; 12: 277–88.
4. Obwegeser H. Surgery of the maxilla for the correction of prognathism. SSO Schweiz Monatsschr Zahnheilkd. 1965; 75: 365–74.
5. Bell WH. Revascularization and bone healing after posterior maxillary osteotomy. J Oral Surg. 1969; 27: 249–55.
6. Bell WH, Levy, BM. Revascularization and bone healing after posterior maxillary osteotomy. J Oral Surg. 1973; 29: 313–20.
7. Bell WH. Biologic basis for maxillary osteotomies. Am J Phys Anthropol. 1973; 38: 279–89.
8. Nelson R, Path, MG, Ogle RG, et al. Quantitation of blood flow after anterior maxillary osteotomy: investigation of 3 surgical approaches. J Oral Surg. 1978; 36: 106–11.
9. Quejada J, Kawamura H, Finn RA, Bell WH. Wound healing associated with segmental total maxillary osteotomy. J Oral Maxillofac Surg. 1986; 44: 366–77.
10. Justus T, Chang BL, Bloomquist D, Ramsay DS. Human gingival and pulpal blood flow during healing after Le Fort I osteotomy. J Oral Maxillofac Surg. 2001; 59: 2–7.
11. Thomas BD, Robert AB, Michael CN. Maxillary perfusion during Le Fort I osteotomy after ligation of the descending palatine artery. J Oral Maxillofac Surg. 1997; 55: 51–5.
12. Epker BN. Vascular considerations in orthognathic surgery. II. Maxillary osteotomies. J Oral Surg. 1984; 57: 473–8.

13. Lanigan DT, Hey JH, West RA. Aseptic necrosis following maxillary osteotomies: report of 36 cases. J Oral Maxillofac Surg. 1990; 48: 142–56.
14. Posnick JC, Tompson B. Cleft-orthognathic surgery. Complications and long-term results. Plas Recon Surg. 1995; 96: 255–66.
15. James DR, Brook, K. Maxillary hypoplasia in patients with cleft lip and palate defortmity – the alternative surgical approach. Eur J Orthodon. 1985; 7: 231–47.
16. Ellis E, Zide, MF. Approaches to the maxilla. In Ellis E, Zide MF (Eds.): Surgical Approaches to the Facial Skeleton. Philadelphia: Lippincott Williams & Wilkins, 2006.

CHAPTER 6

Human Papillomavirus and Survival of Patients with Oropharyngeal Cancer

Ang KK, Harris J, Wheeler R, et al. N Engl J Med.
2010; 363: 24–35.

Reviewed by Andrew Schache

Research Question/Objective

By the start of the 2000s, it was clear that human papillomavirus (HPV)-positive oropharyngeal squamous cell carcinoma (OPSCC) was a distinct entity in terms of aetiology, molecular biology, and clinicopathological presentation[1-3] when compared to non-HPV-related OPSCC.

Evidence of differential survival for HPV-positive OPSCC was found in several case series[4] and a prospective study,[5] but sample size and other limitations restricted a firm conclusion that HPV status alone accounted for prognostic advantage rather than merely patient-related characteristics.

Ang and colleagues[6] sought to provide definitive evidence of the influence of HPV status on survival in patients with OPSCC from a prospective study with adequate sample size.

Study Design

Retrospective analysis of tumour HPV status and survival from patients recruited to a randomised control trial (RTOG 0129) designed to compare accelerated-fractionation radiotherapy (and cisplatin) with standard-fractional radiotherapy (and cisplatin) in the management of stage III or IV Head & Neck SCC.

HPV tumour status determination was a post hoc analysis and was restricted to those patients with tumours arising within the oropharynx. Formalin-fixed paraffin-embedded (FFPE) tumour specimens were assessed for evidence of viral DNA presence (HPV DNA in situ hybridisation, or ISH) and importantly also cellular response to viral oncogene expression through analysis of p16 immunohistochemistry (IHC).

The RTOG 0129 endpoints were overall survival (OS; primary endpoint) and progression-free survival (PFS, secondary endpoint).

Sample Size

721 patients meeting the protocol inclusion criteria were enrolled to RTOG 0129, of whom 60.1% (433/721) had OPSCC. Tumour HPV status was determined in 74.6% (323/433) of OPSCC cases.

Follow-up

Trial patients were seen every 3 months for the first 2 years, every 6 months from years 3 to 5, and annually thereafter.

Inclusion/Exclusion Criteria

Retrospective (post hoc) analysis of trial (RTOG 0129) patients with OPSCC for whom tumour tissue was available for HPV status determination. Lifetime tobacco exposure was collected by standardised, self-administered questionnaire at trial enrollment.

Original trial inclusion criteria:

- Treatment naïve, pathologically confirmed, stage III or IV squamous cell carcinoma of the oral cavity, oropharynx, hypopharynx or larynx with distant metastases (M0)
- Zubrod's performance status (0,1) with adequate bone marrow, hepatic and renal function
- Age ≥18 years

Intervention or Treatment Received

High-dose cisplatin concurrently with either accelerated-fractionation radiotherapy, 72 Gy in 42 fractions over 6 weeks (with concomitant boost of twice-daily irradiation for 12 treatment days), or standardised-fractionation radiotherapy, 70 Gy in 30 fractions over a 7-week period. Cisplatin dosing was calculated at a rate of 100 mg per metre square of body surface area (on days 1 and 22 and days 1, 22, and 43 in accelerated-fractional and standardised-fractionation radiotherapy groups, respectively.

Results

HPV status was determined for 323/422 OPSCC within the trial. There were no significant differences in clinicopathological or survival outcomes between cases with tumour available for HPV status determination and those for which it was not.

Of the 323 OPSCC cases for which HPV status was determined, 206 (63.8%) were positive for HPV DNA (HPV DNA ISH); of these, the vast majority (192/206, 93.2%) were also p16 ISH positive.

Characteristics: Individuals with HPV-positive tumours were statistically more likely to be younger, white, nonsmokers, and have smaller T-stage primary tumours. The two treatment were well balanced with respect to HPV status.

Survival: Overall and progression-free survival was substantially better among patients with HPV-positive tumours than HPV negative counterparts ($p < 0.001$ for both endpoints by log-rank test).

OS at 3 years was 82.4% (95% CI, 77.2–87.6) for patients with HPV-positive OPSCC and 57.1% (95% CI, 48.1–66.1) for patients with HPV negative cancers.

Despite adjustment for other significant determinants of survival (age, race, performance status, smoking, and disease stage) following multivariant analysis, patients with HPV-positive OPSCC still had demonstrably reduced (58%) risk of death as compared to HPV negative (HR, 0.42; 95% CI, 0.27–0.66).

Smoking was also an independent determinant of outcome (OS and PFS) in both HPV-positive and -negative OPSCC. Recursive-partitioning analysis demonstrated HPV status to be the major determinant of survival followed by number of smoking pack-years and advancing nodal stage (in HPV-positive tumours) and advancing tumour stage (in HPV negative disease). Interestingly, the other (non-HPV) favourable prognostic indicators still only explained 10% of apparent survival differences.

Patients with OPSCC were classified into three categories (high, intermediate, and low risk of death) using recursive-partitioning analysis to identify the most influential prognostic factors; subsequently referred to by some as "The Good, The Bad, and The Ugly of OPSCC."

HPV-positive OPSCC patients were considered to be low risk unless they possessed high nodal burden or had >10 pack-year tobacco history, which placed them into an intermediate risk group along with HPV negative OPSCC patients who had less advanced tumour stage (T2-3) and low tobacco exposure (<10-year pack history). High-risk patients had more advanced (T4) HPV negative disease and a >10 pack-year tobacco history.

Study Limitations

Although this work represents a defining point in the understanding of HPV-related OPSCC, there are some limitations to the publication. The impact of smoking is relevant; however, caution should be exercised when considering smoking data, as its reporting is notoriously inaccurate even in trial settings (misrepresentation propensity).

The assessment of HPV status in the OPSCC cases recruited to RTOG 0129 was a post hoc analysis (not part of the original study protocol) and only two-thirds of cases had tissue available for HPV status assessment. While there were no significant differences in patient demographics or outcomes between those with or those without tissue, a potential for selection bias remains.

Relevant Studies

Ang et al.[6] provided a clear incentive to seek clinical trial-based modification (deescalation) of therapeutic intensity in HPV-positive OSPCC seeking to reduce the morbidity of treatment and preserve survival benefit. Trials such as RTOG 1016[7] and De-ESCALaTE[8] followed, comparing concomitant cisplatin and radiotherapy, against cetuximab bio-radiotherapy. Interestingly, both found in in favour of cisplatin chemoradiotherapy (CRT), the current standard of care for nonsurgical management of HPV-positive OSPCC.

Advances in surgical technologies and techniques have offered the potential to explore treatment deintensification for surgically managed HPV-positive OPSCC with the aim of abrogating the functional and quality of life implications of primary CRT. Trials such as ECOG 3311[9] and PATHOS[10] utilise transoral robotic surgery and/or transoral laser microsurgery for this purpose. On the basis of resective pathology including stage, nodal status, evidence of extracapsular spread (now termed extranodal extension), and surgical margins, these trials apply surgically based risk stratification, allocating patients to adjuvant therapy with randomisation in each arm including deintensified therapeutic alternatives.

A pressing need still remains to explore the reasons for treatment failure in the relatively small group of HPV-positive individuals with poorest outcomes (both intermediate- and low-risk groups). Their identification remains a priority as the clinical and academic community continues to explore alterations to treatment paradigms, such that we might avoid potentially catastrophic outcomes of treatment deintensification in these individuals.

The prognostic significance of HPV status, evidenced by Ang et al.,[6] has recently been recognised in the revised AJCC tumour staging classification[11] such that a separate staging algorithm now exists for HPV-positive OPSCC distinguishing it from tumours with other causes (albeit utilising only single modality testing; p16 immunochemistry).

REFERENCES

1. Gillison ML, Koch WM, Capone RB, et al. Evidence for a causal association between human papillomavirus and a subset of head and neck cancers. J Natl Cancer Inst. 2000; 92: 709–20.

2. Gillison ML, D'Souza G, Westra W, et al. Distinct risk factor profiles for human papillomavirus type 16-positive and human papillomavirus type 16-negative head and neck cancers. J Natl Cancer Inst. 2008; 100: 407–20.

3. D'Souza G, Kreimer AR, Viscidi R, et al. Case-control study of human papillomavirus and oropharyngeal cancer. N Engl J Med. 2007; 356: 1944–56.

4. Ragin CC, Taioli E. Survival of squamous cell carcinoma of the head and neck in relation to human papillomavirus infection: review and meta-analysis. Int J Cancer. 2007; 121: 1813–20.

5. Fakhry C, Westra WH, Li S, et al. Improved survival of patients with human papillomavirus-positive head and neck squamous cell carcinoma in a prospective clinical trial. J Natl Cancer Inst. 2008; 100: 261–9.

6. Ang KK, Harris J, Wheeler R, et al. Human papillomavirus and survival of patients with oropharyngeal cancer. N Engl J Med. 2010; 363: 24–35.

7. Gillison ML, Trotti AM, Harris J, et al. Radiotherapy plus cetuximab or cisplatin in human papillomavirus-positive oropharyngeal cancer (NRG Oncology RTOG 1016): a randomised, multicentre, non-inferiority trial. Lancet. 2019; 393: 40–50.

8. Mehanna H, Robinson M, Hartley A, et al. Radiotherapy plus cisplatin or cetuximab in low-risk human papillomavirus-positive oropharyngeal cancer (De-ESCALaTE HPV): an open-label randomised controlled phase 3 trial. Lancet. 2019; 393: 51–60.

9. Transoral surgery followed by low-dose or standard-dose radiation therapy with or without chemotherapy in treating patients with HPV positive stage III–IVA oropharyngeal cancer. [Available from: https://clinicaltrials.gov/ct2/show/NCT01898494.]

10. Owadally W, Hurt C, Timmins H, et al. PATHOS: a phase II/III trial of risk-stratified, reduced intensity adjuvant treatment in patients undergoing transoral surgery for human papillomavirus (HPV) positive oropharyngeal cancer. BMC Cancer. 2015; 15: 602.

11. Edge SB. (Ed.). AJCC Cancer Staging Manual, 8th ed. New York: Springer, 2017.

CHAPTER 7

Analysis of 49 Cases of Flap Compromise in 1,310 Free Flaps for Head and Neck Reconstruction

Yu P, Chang DW, Miller MJ, Reece G, Robb GL. Head Neck. 2009; 31: 45–51.

Reviewed by Alasdair McKechnie

Research Question/Objective

The experience was presented of free flap reconstruction of head and neck defects at the M.D. Anderson Cancer Center over an 11-year period from 1995 to 2006, The authors described rates of flap compromise, salvage, and failure and analysed factors that may contribute to the risk of a poor outcome. Particular attention was paid to technical operative errors and whether the experience of surgeons can predict the likelihood of complications.

Study Design

Retrospective review of 1,310 free flap reconstructions for head and neck defects in a single centre over 11 years.

Sample Size

In 1,266 patients, 1,310 free flaps were performed, including 31 pairs of double flaps and 13 free flaps performed following loss of an earlier reconstruction.

Follow-up

Flap compromise or failure was described in terms of time following surgery up to 7 days. Flap failures occurring after 7 days were grouped together and exact follow-up periods were not given.

Inclusion/Exclusion Criteria

All patients undergoing free flap reconstruction of head and neck defects between 1995 and 2006 were included. Data on causes and factors related to flap compromise were collected. Patients with intraoperative thrombosis that was revised without further consequences were not included in the group of compromised or failed flaps. Analysis of flap compromise and failure rates for full-time faculty members who joined the centre during the study period was performed.

Intervention or Treatment Received

Patients underwent free flap reconstruction of head and neck defects and were managed according to the centre's standard perioperative care routine. Demographic data, site of reconstruction, and previous radiotherapy were recorded. The timing of flap compromise, associated technical factors, and outcomes were also analysed. The surgeons involved in the study were a group of 22 surgeons, including 10 full-time surgeons who commenced their faculty membership during the study period. The relationship between surgeons' microvascular experience and complication rate was explored.

Results

Forty-nine flaps (3.7%) developed signs of vascular compromise. Arterial occlusion (12 flaps) tended to occur early and was more frequently associated with intraoperative difficulties such as thrombosis or atheroma/calcification of the pedicle vessel. While venous compromise was more frequent (31 flaps), it was more likely to be salvageable (58% vs. 33%) than arterial compromise. In six cases of late failure, it was not possible to tell whether the underlying cause was arterial or venous. The overall flap failure rate was 2%.

Female patients were found to be at higher risk of flap failure (OR 2.11, 95% CI, 1.19–3.74, $p = 0.011$), but the authors proposed that this finding be interpreted with caution. Forty-four percent of the flaps were performed in patients who had been previously treated with radiotherapy, and the rates of flap compromise and failure were comparable for irradiated and non-irradiated sites.

In considering the effect of surgical experience on rates of complications, no direct correlation was found, but surgeons who had greater experience did appear to be a more homogeneous group in this respect. When rates of compromise and failure were compared in two groups of surgeons, those who performed 70 procedures or more had significantly lower rates of both flap compromise and flap loss (Figure 7.1).

Study Limitations

Clearly a prospective randomised trial would not be appropriate in this context. Selection bias may therefore have skewed the results of this study. The authors admitted that the rate of flap compromise and loss was too low to allow meaningful analysis of predisposing factors, a fact that might allow the authors a deserved sense of satisfaction! While the results of this study set a benchmark for success in free flap reconstruction, the paper lacked detail in a number of key areas. The site of reconstruction was reported, but donor sites were not. The authors alluded to an increase in the number of anterolateral thigh (ALT) flaps towards the end of the study period, but no further detail was provided. While the authors did consider the effect of preoperative radiotherapy on flap compromise rates, they did not include detail on whether the subsequent

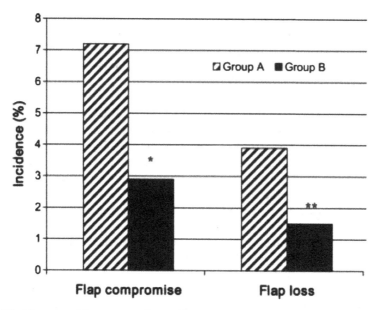

Figure 7.1 The rates of flap compromise and failure among surgeons who performed fewer than 70 free flaps (groups A) and more than 70 free flaps (groups B) during the 11-year time period. $*p = 0.007$; $**p = 0.04$.

reconstruction was being performed as part of a planned combined modality treatment or as a salvage procedure for recurrence. Furthermore, no information on adjuvant chemotherapy was included in the analysis.

The study also compared flap compromise and flap failure rates between groups of surgeons with differing levels of experience. It is unclear how prior experience was defined: did "performed" mean the surgeon harvested the tissue, inset the flap, or completed one or more anastomoses?

Relevant Studies

This paper remains one of the largest published series of free flap reconstructions for head and neck cancer and marks a "coming of age" for head and neck surgery. Over the preceding decades, microvascular techniques had been first developed and then adapted for oral and pharyngeal reconstruction.[1–3] Unsurprisingly, early reports reflected a pioneering but cautious approach. Refinement of the existing methods and development of newer techniques brought greater confidence and larger published series of free flaps.[4–6]

With improved experience, clinicians were able to define standards and study the factors that might influence success rates and complications. Urken et al. analysed complications in a series of 200 microvascular reconstructions, half of which were performed for recurrent disease or secondary reconstruction.

Radiotherapy prior to surgery was cited as a factor in recipient site wound breakdown, but no further statistical analysis was provided. Keiner et al. reported a smaller series with better overall flap success rates in the irradiated group[7,8], and an earlier paper from MD Anderson also showed no adverse effect on flap survival with prior radiotherapy.[9]

A more recent report from the same institution described a series of patients treated between 2000 and 2010, presumably including some of the same patients who were included in Yu's paper. In this series of 2,296 flaps, prior radiotherapy was not associated with flap failure but chemotherapy was.[10] Perhaps reflecting the division of responsibility within the authors' institutions, these papers have tended to focus on success of the microvascular reconstruction. Patients with head and neck cancer frequently have comorbidities and an arguably more appropriate approach is to analyse risk factors for all systemic and local complications. McMahon et al. has published two detailed studies that help put flap compromise and flap failure in context.[11,12]

The learning curve associated with developing a reconstructive practice has been analysed by other authors. Kim et al. compared free flap compromise and failure rate in the first 150 cases performed by the team rather than concentrating on individual experience, demonstrating improved outcomes with increased experience.[13] Brady et al. analysed a large group of patients treated in multiple centres.[14] The involvement of trainees and their level of training was included, but their exact role in the surgery was not clarified. This study showed an inverse correlation between the level of experience of the trainee and the length of operation but no effect on flap failure.

This paper is arguably as important for the incidental information on the institutional infrastructure associated with a successful high-volume reconstructive practice as for the results of the analysis. The use of a dedicated intensive care facility and "flap floor" solely for the purpose of postoperative care of reconstruction patients, highly experienced nursing staff, and ease of access to theatres that allows a reliable return to theatre within 1 to 2 hours of suspected flap compromise are all indicative of an institutional dedication to high-quality care.

REFERENCES

1. MacLeod AM, O'Brien BM, Morrison WA. Microvascular techniques in reconstruction following major resections for cancer of the head and neck. Aust N Z J Surg. 1979; 49: 648–53.
2. Soutar DS, Scheker LR, Tanner NS, McGregor IA. The radial forearm flap: a versatile method for intra-oral reconstruction. Br J Plast Surg. 1983; 36: 1–8.
3. Takato T, Harii K, Ebihara S, et al. Oral and pharyngeal reconstruction using the free forearm flap. Arch Otolaryngol Head Neck Surg. 1987; 113: 873–9.

4. Schusterman MA, Miller MJ, Reece GP, et al. A single center's experience with 308 free flaps for repair of head and neck cancer defects. Plast Reconstr Surg. 1994; 93: 472–8; discussion 479–80.

5. O'Brien CJ, Lee KK, Stern HS, et al. Evaluation of 250 free-flap reconstructions after resection of tumours of the head and neck. Aust N Z J Surg. 1998; 68: 698–701.

6. Nakatsuka T, Harii K, Asato H, et al. Analytic review of 2372 free flap transfers for head and neck reconstruction following cancer resection. J Reconstr Microsurg. 2003; 19: 363–8; discussion 9.

7. Kiener JL, Hoffman WY, Mathes SJ. Influence of radiotherapy on microvascular reconstruction in the head and neck region. Am J Surg. 1991; 162: 404–7.

8. Urken ML, Weinberg H, Buchbinder D, et al. Microvascular free flaps in head and neck reconstruction. Report of 200 cases and review of complications. Arch Otolaryngol Head Neck Surg. 1994; 120: 633–40.

9. Bengtson BP, Schusterman MA, Baldwin BJ, et al. Influence of prior radiotherapy on the development of postoperative complications and success of free tissue transfers in head and neck cancer reconstruction. Am J Surg. 1993; 166: 326–30.

10. Chang EI, Zhang H, Liu J, et al. Analysis of risk factors for flap loss and salvage in free flap head and neck reconstruction. Head Neck. 2016; 38: E771–5.

11. McMahon JD, MacIver C, Smith M, et al. Postoperative complications after major head and neck surgery with free flap repair–prevalence, patterns, and determinants: a prospective cohort study. Br J Oral Maxillofac Surg. 2013; 51: 689–95.

12. McMahon J, Handley TPB, Bobinskas A, et al. Postoperative complications after head and neck operations that require free tissue transfer – prevalent, morbid, and costly. Br J Oral Maxillofac Surg. 2017; 55: 809–14.

13. Kim H, Jeong WJ, Ahn SH. Results of free flap reconstruction after ablative surgery in the head and neck. Clin Exp Otorhinolaryngol. 2015; 8: 167–73.

14. Brady JS, Crippen MM, Filimonov A, et al. The effect of training level on complications after free flap surgery of the head and neck. Am J Otolaryngol. 2017; 38: 560–4.

CHAPTER 8

Postoperative Irradiation with or without Concomitant Chemotherapy for Locally Advanced Head and Neck Cancer

Bernier J, Domenge C, Ozsahin M, et al. European Organization for Research and Treatment of Cancer Trial 22931. N Engl J Med. 2004; 350: 1945–52.

Reviewed by Stergios Doumas and Anastasios Kanatas

Research Question/Objective

The authors compared radiotherapy and chemoradiotherapy (cisplatin with radiotherapy) as adjuvant treatments following surgery for stage III or IV head and neck squamous cell carcinoma (HNSCC).

Study Design

Multicentre prospective randomised phase III trial by the EORTC Data Centre, including patients with stage III–IV operable HNSCC. After undergoing resection and neck dissection, 167 patients were randomly assigned to receive radiotherapy alone and 167 to receive the same radiotherapy (XRT) regimen combined with 3 cycles of cisplatin on days 1, 22, and 43 of the radiotherapy regimen (CRT).

Primary endpoints: Progression free survival (PFS) and overall survival (OS) were estimated by Kaplan-Meier curves. Both parameters were evaluated from the time of randomisation to the time of progression of the disease/or death, and death, respectively.

Secondary Endpoints

Cumulative incidences of local or regional relapses, late reactions, metastases, and second primary tumours. The trial was designed to detect an absolute increase in PFS of 15% (from 40% to 55% at 3 years) with a two-sided 5% significance level and a statistical power of 80%.

Sample Size

From February 1994 to October 2000, 334 patients from 23 institutions consented to participate in the trial; 92% were men and 69% were more than

50 years of age. These patients were randomly allocated into two groups involving X-ray radiotherapy (XRT) and carbon-ion radiotherapy (CRT), respectively. The baseline characteristics of the two groups were similar in sex, age, tumour stage, nodal stage, primary tumour site, resection margin status, histological differentiation, extracapsular spread, perineural invasion, vascular embolisms, and lymph node involvement.

Follow-up

The median and maximal follow-up times were 60 months and 100 months, respectively. Patients were evaluated every 2 months for the first 6 months, every 4 months for the next 24 months, every 6 months for the next 2 years, and annually thereafter.

Inclusion Criteria

- Consent form obtained
- Histologically confirmed squamous cell carcinoma (SCC), previously untreated, of the oral cavity, oropharynx, hypopharynx or larynx, of tumours (T) pathological stage pT3 or pT4, and any nodal (N) stage without distal metastasis (M0)
- Any tumour of the above subsites of pT1 or pT2 and N2 or N3, M0 stage
- pT1 or pT2 and N0, N1, M0 stage tumours with adverse features (ECS, positive margins, PNI, LVI)
- Oral cavity or oropharyngeal tumours with involved nodes at level IV or V as per Robbins classification
- Age: 18–70 years
- Performance Status (PS) 0–2
- Serum creatinine ≤ 120 µmol/L (1.36 mg/dL)
- WCC ≥ 4,000/mm³
- Platelets ≥ 100,000/mm³
- Hb ≥ 11.0 g/dL
- ALT, AST, bilirubin ≤ 2 × institutional upper limit of normal

Exclusion Criteria

- pT3 N0 laryngeal SCC
- History of invasive or synchronous cancer (except nonmelanoma skin cancer)
- Previously received chemotherapy
- Known central nervous system disease

Intervention or Treatment Received

All 334 patients had surgery with curative intent. Of these, 167 patients were randomly assigned to receive XRT alone and 167 to receive the same

XRT regimen combined with 100 mg/m^2 cisplatin on days 1, 22 and 43 of the XRT regimen. A large volume encompassing the primary site and all draining lymph nodes at risk received a dose of up to 54 Gy in 27 fractions over a period of 5 1/2 weeks. Regions that were at high risk for malignant dissemination or that had inadequate resection margins (<5 mm) received a 12-Gy boost (total, 66 Gy) in 33 fractions over a period of 6 1/2 weeks. The dose to the spinal cord was limited to 45 Gy.

Results

The 5-year PFS and OS were 36% versus 47% (HR 0.75; 95% CI, 0.56–0.99), and 40% versus 53% ($p = 0.02$, HR for death 0.70, 95% CI, 0.52–0.95) between the XRT and CRT group, respectively.

In line with this, the estimated 5-year cumulative incidence for locoregional recurrence was 31% versus 18% ($p = 0.007$), respectively. The risk of distant metastasis and second primaries was not statistically significant. Equally, the rate of late complications seemed to be comparable. However, fibrosis was more prominent in the CRT group, but xerostomia was worse in the XRT group.

Study Limitations

This study showed that the adjuvant CRT confers survival benefit in stage III–IV HNSCC in terms of OS and PFS, but it seems that the addition of the radiosensitizer cisplatin failed to improve distal metastasis or second primaries.

There have been issues with patients' chemotherapy tolerability due to toxicity, as 10% never started chemotherapy, 11% stopped after first cycle, and an additional 15% ceased after the second cycle in the aforementioned study.[1] There are have been some grade 3 or higher acute toxicities; such as mucositis, granulocytopenia, leukopenia and vomiting.

The authors also acknowledged that the number of patients per subsite was not as well balanced as in RTOG 9501.[2] Quality of life (QoL) was not assessed.

A major limitation in both studies (EORTC, RTOG) is that they were not stratified per tumour site and HPV status as they were conducted in the pre-HPV OPC era. It is now plausible that this particular group has different biological behaviours. Hence, the TNM 8th edition sub-classifies OPC into p16+ and p16– subgroups. p16 is the best surrogate marker of HPV infection in these tumours.[3] Efforts are also being made to de-escalate treatment in HPV+ OPC.[4]

Relevant Studies

EORTC 22931 and RTOG 9501 provided level I evidence and established the foundations for the administration of concomitant CRT in surgically treated, locally advanced physically fit HNSCC patients with ECS and positive margins.[1,2,5–7] Bernier at al. carried out collaborative comparative analysis of EORTC and RTOG and additionally concluded that there was also a trend in favour of CRT in the group of patients who had stage III–IV disease, PNI, LVI, and/or clinically enlarged level IV–V lymph nodes secondary to tumours arising in the oral cavity or oropharynx.[6] These findings have been adopted by both US NCCN and UK guidelines for surgically treated locally advanced HNSCC.[5,7]

However, RTOG 9501 did not show any benefit in OS (HR 0.84, 95% CI, 0.65–1.09; $P = 0.19$). Akin to EORTC, DFS was significantly longer in the combined-therapy group than in the radiotherapy group (HR for disease or death, 0.78; 95% CI, 0.61–0.99; $P = 0.04$), incidence of acute adverse effects of grade 3 or greater was 34% in the RT group vs 77% in CRT group ($P < 0.001$).[2] In 2012 Cooper et al. presented their 10-y data of RTOG 9501. It is noteworthy that at 9.4 years there was no long-term benefit for the addition of concurrent cisplatin to postoperative RT for the primary endpoint of locoregional control or the secondary endpoints of DFS and OS for all eligible randomised patients. However, significant improvements in locoregional control and DFS from concurrent cisplatin persisted in the subgroup that had ECS and/or involved margins.[8]

In 2009, Rosenthal et al. presented the results of RTOG 0024, a phase II trial involving early postoperative paclitaxel followed by concurrent paclitaxel and cisplatin as CRT in post-resected locally advanced HNSCC in 70 patients with aggressive tumour features (positive margins, ECS, multiple positive nodes).[9] It was found to be a well-tolerated regime and their survival benefits were superior to RTOG 9501 for this particular patient subgroup (estimated 2-year locoregional failure rate 12%, 95% CI, 47.5%–71.5%, 2-year OS 64.7%, 95% CI, 52.8%–76.6%).[9]

More recently, Harari et al. conducted the RTOG 0234, a phase II randomised trial. Eligibility required pathologic stage III to IV SCCHN with gross total resection showing positive margins and/or extracapsular nodal extension and/or two or more nodal metastases. Patients were randomly assigned to 60 Gy radiation with cetuximab once per week plus either low-dose cisplatin or docetaxel once per week. Again, this regime was well tolerated and 2-year OS was superior (especially the docetaxel subgroup) to RTOG 9501.[10]

Immunotherapy is an emerging modality for cancer treatment with a role in recurrent/metastatic HNSCC setting. However, its role in the locally advanced HNSCC as upfront or adjuvant treatment is under scrutiny.[11–13]

REFERENCES

1. Bernier J, Domenge C, Ozsahin M, et al. Postoperative irradiation with or without concomitant chemotherapy for locally advanced head and neck cancer. European organization for research and treatment of cancer trial 22931. N Engl J Med. 2004; 350: 1945–52.
2. Cooper JS, Pajak TF, Forastiere AA, et al. Postoperative concurrent radiotherapy and chemotherapy for high-risk squamous-cell carcinoma of the head and neck. N Engl J Med. 2004; 350: 1937–44.
3. Lydiatt WM, Patel SG, O'Sullivan B, et al. Head and neck cancers—major changes in the American Joint Committee on cancer eighth edition cancer staging manual. CA Cancer J Clin. 2017; 67: 122–37.
4. Kirtane K, Rodriguez CP. Postoperative combined modality treatment in high risk resected locally advanced squamous cell carcinomas of the head and neck (HNSCC). Front Oncol. 2018; 8: 588.
5. National Comprehensive Cancer Network Guidelines for Head & Neck Cancers. Available from: https://www.nccn.org/store/login/login.aspx?ReturnURL=https://www.nccn.org/professionals/physician_gls/PDF/head-and-neck.pdf. Accessed 8/12/2018.
6. Bernier J, Cooper JS, Pajak TF, et al. Defining risk levels in locally advanced head and neck cancers: a comparative analysis of concurrent postoperative radiation plus chemotherapy trials of the EORTC (#22931) and RTOG (# 9501). Head Neck. 2005; 27: 843–50.
7. Paleri V, Urbano TG, Mehanna H, et al. Management of neck metastases in head and neck cancer: United Kingdom National Multidisciplinary Guidelines. J Laryngol Otol. 2016; 130: S161–9.
8. Cooper JS, Zhang Q, Pajak TF, et al. Long-term follow-up of the RTOG 9501/intergroup phase III trial: postoperative concurrent radiation therapy and chemotherapy in high-risk squamous cell carcinoma of the head and neck. Int J Radiat Oncol Biol Phys. 2012; 84: 1198–205.
9. Rosenthal DI, Harris J, Forastiere AA, et al. Early postoperative paclitaxel followed by concurrent paclitaxel and cisplatin with radiation therapy for patients with resected high-risk head and neck squamous cell carcinoma: report of the phase II trial RTOG 0024. J Clin Oncol. 2009; 27: 4727–32.
10. Harari PM, Harris J, Kies MS, et al. Postoperative chemoradiotherapy and cetuximab for high-risk squamous cell carcinoma of the head and neck: Radiation Therapy Oncology Group RTOG-0234. J Clin Oncol. 2014; 32: 2586–95.
11. Sim F, Leidner R, Bell RB. Immunotherapy for head and neck cancer. Oral Maxillofac Surg Clin North Am. 2019; 31: 85–100.
12. Hanna GJ, Adkins DR, Zolkind P, Uppaluri R. Rationale for neoadjuvant immunotherapy in head and neck squamous cell carcinoma. Oral Oncol. 2017; 73: 65–9.
13. Economopoulou P, Kotsantis I, Psyrri A. The promise of immunotherapy in head and neck squamous cell carcinoma: combinatorial immunotherapy approaches. ESMO Open. 2017; 1: e000122.

CHAPTER 9

The Patterns of Cervical Lymph Node Metastasis from Squamous Cell Carcinoma of the Oral Cavity

Jatin Shah J, Candela F, Podder A. Cancer. 1990; 66: 109–13.

Reviewed by Jag Dhanda and Raghuram Boyapati

Research Question/Objective

The prevalence and distribution of cervical metastasis in oral cavity squamous cell carcinoma (OSCC).

Study Design

A consecutive series of 501 previously untreated patients undergoing a radical neck dissection (RND) for OSCC. In this retrospective analysis, patients were subclassified by the clinical node status N0 or N+ and three neck dissection (ND) treatment groups: elective dissection (ED) for patients with a clinically N0 neck, a therapeutic or immediate therapeutic dissection (ITD) for patients with cervical metastasis (N+), or subsequent therapeutic dissection (STD) for salvage (N+) cases with initially conservative management of the neck and subsequent relapse with cervical metastasis (N+).

Sample Size

A total of 501 previously treated patients between December 1965 and December 1986. Of these, 192 ED patients, 206 ITD, and 103 STD patients.

Follow-up

Mean time for relapse for the STD group was 7 months; long-term follow-up not stated.

Inclusion/Exclusion Criteria

Inclusion criteria–Histological SCC including variants such as verrucous and spindle cell with patients having an immediate or delayed RND.

Exclusion criteria–Lip primary, partial neck dissection, multiple primaries, preoperative chemotherapy, preoperative radiation therapy, or inadequate data.

Intervention or Treatment Received

RND with or without primary site OSCC resection.

Results

1. Distribution by site–Oral tongue 36% and FOM 33%, gingiva 21%, retromolar trigone 5%, cheek 5% and hard palate 1%
2. Distribution by clinical stage–Stage I 19%, stage II 29%, stage III 36% and stage IV 16%
3. Distribution of ND groups–ED 192 (38%), ITD 206 (41%) and STD 103 (21%)
4. Prevalence of nodal metastasis in ND groups—ED 34% (occult metastasis), ITD 69%, STD 90%
5. Prevalence of nodal metastasis by neck level
   a. Level V prevalence very low regardless of treatment intent (<4%) with 6% positive for FOM and gingiva in ITD group and 12% FOM positive in STD group; all these patients were positive at all other levels
   b. Level IV prevalence
      i. ED 3%, 15% ITD and 16% STD
      ii. Subsite involvement ED ranging from 2 to 6% with 50% of cases with isolated level involvement, ITD range 7–29% with tongue (21%) and RMT (29%) highest, STD 20% original tongue primaries
   c. Level III sharp increase involvement for N+ groups
      i. ED 9%, ITD 31% and 39% STD
      ii. Subsite involvement ED 16% tongue and 7% FOM, ITD 38% tongue 34% FOM and 29% RMT, STD 66% RMT, 50% cheek, 45% tongue
   d. Levels I and II
      i. Levels I and II highest rates of metastasis (42% and 54%, respectively)
      ii. Increasing rates for ED (20% and 17%), ITD (48% and 38%), and STD (42% and 54%) for levels I and II, respectively
      iii. All subsites found for ED, ITD, and STD, the less common subsites, such as RMT, gum and cheek, were more likely to involve upper levels of neck than lower levels of neck.
6. Accuracy of clinical examination at best approximately two-thirds (ED 70%, ITD 65% and STD 68%) and level IV very poor (20%)

Study Limitations

A retrospective study with limited methodology on pathology sample analysis (step serial section) and lacking detail for justification or indication of ED in N0 cases; it was presumed by the authors that these cases "represented increased risk of harbouring micrometastasis in the judgment of the surgeon."

Relevant Studies

This study was part of a larger series of 1,081 patients undergoing 1,119 RNDs for SCC of the upper aerodigestive tract.[1] Primary tumours were oropharynx (207 patients), hypopharynx (126 patients) and larynx (247 patients) with the findings for oral cavity involvement (501 patients) published in more detail in this additional paper. The most significant findings of these two papers were presence of micrometastasis (or occult metastasis) in one-third of cases and the tendency for certain levels of the neck to be involved depending upon the primary site. This paper showed that levels I, II, and III were at higher risk of metastasis from oral cavity disease whereas levels II, III, and IV were at higher risk from carcinomas of the oropharynx, hypopharynx, and larynx. The two papers led to the recommendation of a supraomohyoid ND (levels I–III) for the N0 or early disease with a primary oral cavity SCC and an anterolateral ND (levels II–IV) for N0 or early disease patients with primary SCC of the oropharynx, hypopharynx and larynx.

The paper was an important milestone in the development of the neck dissection, a procedure which has been studied for well over 100 years. The first significant published series of en-bloc radical dissection in the management of cervical metastasis in head and neck cancer was the RND first described by Crile in 1906.[2]

The second milestone was the paper by Hayes Martin, chief of the head and neck service at Memorial Hospital, New York, who analysed 1,450 NDs performed from 1928 to 1950.[3] This advocated that the spinal accessory nerve, internal jugular vein and sternocleidomastoid muscle should be removed in the N+ neck. Although sacrificing the accessory nerve was claimed to be the only method of ensuring adequate clearance of level V, and that this would affect the patients' quality of life, this approach became the mainstay of treatment for decades.

By the 1960s, increasing numbers of surgeons including Bocca from Italy and Ballantyne from MD Anderson felt that this radical approach of removing non-lymphatic structures was too morbid for early disease (N1), leading to the modified radical and functional approaches in ND.[4–6] Professor Oswalso Suarez, from Argentina, was the first to introduce the concept of the functional ND in which all the important anatomical structures in the neck could be preserved by removing the cervical fascia, or the aponeurotic envelope, containing the accompanying lymphatics of the neck. In 1984, Bocca demonstrated the oncological safety of the functional neck dissection in 1,200 neck dissections for 843 patients in which he showed a low recurrence rate with improvements in the quality of life.[7]

The selective ND was a further evolution of the procedure, and Shah's paper played a pivotal part in the understanding of the pattern of spread of head and neck malignancy to cervical LNs with the adoption of a more targeted or individualised approach in the management of the neck. This was published at a time when then was increasing momentum for a less functionally and aesthetically morbid procedure.

Although Byers had demonstrated that a modified ND in early disease (N0 or N1) with a supraomohyoid dissection (levels I-III), with or without radiotherapy, showed no difference in outcomes with patients undergoing a functional ND, his work was based on a limited series of patients.[8] Shah's study provided much more substantial evidence with a much larger cohort, but he also looked at the various subsites of the oral cavity as well as the distribution of disease. His analysis provided much more convincing evidence for an algorithm for the management of cervical metastasis.

Shah demonstrated that a supraomohyoid approach in N0 patients would have resulted in seven patients (3.5%) with nodal disease beyond the surgical field (level IV and V), of which three patients had level IV involvement alone. Likewise, if a levels I–IV ND were only performed on N+ cases, 10 patients (3.2%) would have had disease beyond the surgical field involving level V. The standard of care for managing the neck for N0 or early disease is a level I to IV ND, with functional or radical approaches preserved for more advanced disease. This was supported more recently by D'Cruz in his landmark paper in 2015 (see Chapter 10) in which he concluded that the elective neck dissection was superior to watchful waiting for overall and disease-free survival in N0 patients with early oral SCCs.[9]

It is important to be cautious with the interpretation of the findings in this paper for less common subsites of OSCC and the pattern of metastasis. Six percent of retromolar trigone tumours were positive at level IV compared to 3% for the tongue. It is now well established that the tongue carries a higher risk for level IV metastasis, with skip metastasis in levels III and IV described in 16% of cases by Byers.[10] With these low-prevalence sites, even a single case can make a large percentage difference. In Shah's series of retromolar trigone cases (16 patients), just under half were positive (7 patients) with only a single patient positive at level IV. These less frequent sites (cheek, retromolar trigone, and gums) did, however, almost exclusively present with disease in levels I–III.

As well as numerous retrospective studies that followed, in a prospective randomised trial comparing modified RND and SND (I to III) for clinically node-negative patients with T2 to T4 tumours of the oral cavity, the Brazilian Head and Neck Cancer Study Group was unable to show any difference either in 5-year overall survival (OS) or in the rate of neck failure.[11]

In summary, levels I–III are at greatest risk with oral cavity SCC, with level IV rarely involved in N0 disease (3%) and one-third can present with occult disease.

More commonly, level IV is involved in N+ disease (15–16%) and half these patients also have disease in higher levels. Level V is rarely involved in N0 and N+ disease from the oral cavity. The findings supported the move to a selective ND with as suggestion of levels I–III in N0 disease and inclusion of additional levels (IV and V) when intraoperative findings suggest positive disease.

Further evolution of the selective neck dissection has emerged with a new era of super- selective techniques such as sentinel node biopsy for early disease which can further inform the clinician on both ipsilateral and contralateral disease for primary tumours approximating the midline and the need for a neck dissection, while newer techniques in imaging, such as PET-CT, have also increased the specificity of LN assessment.[12–14]

REFERENCES

1. Shah JP. Patterns of cervical lymph node metastasis from squamous carcinomas of the upper aerodigestive tract. Am J Surg. 1990; 160: 405–9.
2. Crile G. Landmark article Dec 1, 1906: excision of cancer of the head and neck. With special reference to the plan of dissection based on one hundred and thirty-two operations. By George Crile. J Am Med Assoc. 1987; 258: 3286–93.
3. Martin H, Del Valle B, Ehrlich H, Cahan WG. Neck dissection. Cancer. 1951; 4: 441–99.
4. Bocca E, Pignataro O. A conservation technique in radical neck dissection. Ann Otol Rhinol Laryngol. 1967; 76: 975–87.
5. Bocca E, Pignataro O, Sasaki CT. Functional neck dissection. A description of operative technique. Arch Otolaryngol. 1980; 106: 524–7.
6. Ballantyne AJ. Neck dissection for cancer. Curr Probl Cancer. 1985; 9: 1–34.
7. Bocca E, Pignataro O, Oldini C, Cappa C. Functional neck dissection: an evaluation and review of 843 cases. Laryngoscope. 1984; 94: 942–5.
8. Byers RM, Wolf PF, Ballantyne AJ. Rationale for elective modified neck dissection. Head Neck Surg. 1988; 10: 160–7.
9. D'Cruz AK, Vaish R, Kapre N, et al. Elective versus therapeutic neck dissection in node-negative Oral cancer. N Engl J Med. 2015; 373: 521–9.
10. Byers RM, Weber RS, Andrews T, et al. Frequency and therapeutic implications of "skip metastases" in the neck from squamous carcinoma of the oral tongue. Head Neck. 1997; 19: 14–9.
11. Brazilian Head and Neck Cancer Study Group. End results of a prospective trial on elective lateral neck dissection vs type III modified radical neck dissection in the management of supraglottic and transglottic carcinomas. Head Neck. 1999; 21: 694–702.
12. Goshen E, Davidson T, Yahalom R, Talmi YP, Zwas ST. PET/CT in the evaluation of patients with squamous cell cancer of the head and neck. Int J Oral Maxillofac Surg. 2006; 35: 332–6.
13. Kim SJ, Pak K, Kim K. Diagnostic accuracy of F-18 FDG PET or PET/CT for detection of lymph node metastasis in clinically node negative head and neck cancer patients: a systematic review and meta-analysis. Am J Otolaryngol. 2019; 40: 297–305.
14. Schilling C, Stoeckli SJ, Vigili MG, et al. Surgical consensus guidelines on sentinel node biopsy (SNB) in patients with oral cancer. Head Neck. 2019; 41: 2655–64.

CHAPTER 10

Tumour Thickness as a Predictor of Nodal Metastases in Oral Cancer: Comparison between Tongue and Floor of Mouth Subsites

Balasubramanian D, Ebrahimi A, Gupta R, et al. Oral Oncol. 2014; 50: 1165–68.

Reviewed by Peyman Alam, Robert Isaac, Tomas Svoboda and Peter A Brennan

Objective/Research Question

To identify whether there is a difference in critical thickness of tongue and floor of mouth (FOM) squamous cell carcinoma (SCC) where the risk of nodal metastasis is high. Results suggested that thin FOM tumours (2.1–4 mm) have a high rate of nodal metastasis, and therefore elective neck dissection (ND) is appropriate in FOM and tongue SCC tumours of greater than 2 mm and 4 mm thickness, respectively.

Study Design

Clinico-pathological data for all patients with oral tongue and FOM SCC treated between 1987 and 2012 in the Department of Head & Neck Surgery, Royal Prince Alfred Hospital (RPAH), Sydney, Australia, was extracted from the database. Maximum tumour thickness was measured on formalin fixed paraffin-embedded sections stained with hematoxylin and eosin to the nearest 0.1 mm using an ocular micrometer. The tumour thickness without superficial keratin and inflammatory debris was measured from the level of adjacent normal mucosa to the deepest point of tumour invasion as described by Moore et al.[1] In this study, the neck was considered positive if either nodal metastasis were proven on elective or therapeutic neck dissection or pathologically proven nodal recurrence occurred during follow-up.

Sample Size

A total of 343 patients were included in this study.

Follow-up

Median follow-up was 2.3 years.

Inclusion/Exclusion Criteria

Patients treated for previous head and neck SCC were excluded.

Intervention or Treatment Received

All 343 patients received wide excision of the primary tumour with curative intend and 262 (76.4%) had neck dissection as part of their initial treatment.

Results

A total of 343 patients were included in this study. There were 227 males and 116 females with a median age of 60 years (range 22–97 years). Out of 262 patients who underwent neck dissection, 188 had an elective ND for clinically N0 disease and 74 had a therapeutic ND for nodal positive disease.

In the FOM group, the majority of patients had an elective neck dissection (73 elective, 34 therapeutic, and 14 had their neck observed). In the tongue cohort, 115 had elective neck dissection for clinically N0 disease, 40 therapeutic neck dissection for N+ disease, and 67 had their neck observed. From the neck observation group (81 patients), 3 received elective neck irradiation and in total 143 patients received radiotherapy due to adverse pathological features.

The FOM group had a higher proportion of patients receiving radiotherapy (52.1% vs. 36.0%, $p = 0.004$).

In patients with a FOM primary tumour thickness of 2.1–4 mm, the rate of nodal metastasis was 41.7%, compared to tongue tumour group with similar thickness, where the rate was only 11.2%. This rate of nodal disease increased to 38.5% in the tongue cancer group with a primary tumour thickness of 4.1–6 mm.

However, the study, did not show an overall statistically significant ($p = 0.21$) increase in nodal metastasis in FOM (44%) compared to the tongue group (37%).

Study Limitations

1. The true neck node positivity can only be appreciated if all the patients included in this study had a neck dissection (which is unethical).
2. The specific tumour thickness cutoffs may not be generalisable.
3. The difference in patients receiving postoperative radiotherapy between the groups may influence the outcome.

Relevant Studies

Nodal metastasis in oral SCC has significant prognostic value, and several primary tumour factors such as tumour size, thickness, and perineural invasion (PNI) have been suggested in relation to development of neck node metastasis.

However, most studies in relation to tumour thickness have predominantly focused on the tongue SCC subsite.

Thiagarajan et al.[2] performed a retrospective study of 586 patients with oral tongue SCC treated primarily by surgery at the Tata Memorial Hospital, Mumbai, between 2007 and 2010, finding that PNI significantly affected disease free survival and a tumour thickness of more than 11 mm significantly affected the overall survival.

Similarly, O Brien et al.[3] measured tumour thickness in 145 oral cavity SCCs, clinically staged as T1 ($n = 62$) or T2 ($n = 83$). Patients were followed up for minimum of 2 years, and thickness was correlated with local control, cervical node involvement, and survival. They concluded that tumour thickness is a highly significant, objectively measurable prognostic factor in early- stage oral cancers. According to this study, prognosis changed significantly at a cutoff of 4 mm with local control, nodal disease, and survival rates.

A consecutive series of 1,081 previously untreated patients undergoing 1,119 radical neck dissections (RNDs) for squamous carcinoma of the head and neck was reviewed by Shah et al. to study the patterns of nodal metastases.[4] Predominance of certain levels was seen for each primary site. Neck levels I, II, and III were at highest risk for metastasis from cancer of the oral cavity, and levels II, III, and IV from carcinomas of the oropharynx, hypopharynx, and larynx. Supraomohyoid neck dissection (clearing levels I, II, and III) for the node negative neck (N0) patients with primary SCC of the oral cavity and anterolateral neck dissection (clearing levels II, III, and IV) for N0 patients with primary SCCs of the oropharynx, hypopharynx, and larynx was recommended.

A similar recommendation was made by Fasunla et al.[5] in a meta-analysis of randomised controlled trials on elective neck dissection versus therapeutic neck dissection in oral cavity cancers with a clinically node-negative (N0) neck. The results showed that elective neck dissection reduced the risk of disease-specific death compared to observation. This is in contrast to a D'Cruz study in 2009[6] which showed no benefit in overall survival following END in N0 patients and therefore suggested the need for a randomised controlled trial. The trial was completed by D'Cruz and published in the New England Journal of Medicine in 2015[7] and is discussed in Chapter 11 of this book.

Finally is a recent published study by Hutchison et al.,[8] who conducted a nationwide randomised trial evaluating selective elective neck dissection for early-stage oral cancer (SEND study). This trial concluded that within a generalisable setting, oral cancer patients who have an upfront END have a lower risk of death/recurrence, even with small tumours.

REFERENCES

1. Moore Kuhns JG, Greenberg RA. Thickness as prognostic aid in upper aerodigestive tract. Cancer-Arch Surg. 1986; 121: 1410–4.
2. Thiagarajan S, Nair S, Nair D, et al. Predictors of prognosis for squamous cell carcinoma of oral tongue. Surg Oncol. 2014; 109: 639–44.
3. O'Brien CJ, Lauer CS, Fredricks S, et al. Tumour thickness influences prognosis of T1 and T2 oral cavity cancer-but what thickness? Head Neck. 2003; 25: 937–45.
4. Shah P. Patterns of cervical lymph node metastasis from squamous carcinomas of the upper aerodigestive tract. Am J Surg. 1990; 160: 405–10.
5. Fasulna AJ, Greene BH, Timmesfeld N, et al. A meta-analysis of the randomized controlled trials on elective neck dissection versus therapeutic neck dissection in oral cavity cancers with clinically node-negative neck. Oral Oncol. 2011; 47: 320–4.
6. D'Cruz A, Ravichand C. Elective neck dissection for the management of the N0 neck in early cancer of the oral tongue: need for a randomized controlled trial. Head Neck. 2009 https://doi.org/10.1002/hed.20988 (conference paper).
7. D'Cruz AK, Vaish R, Kapre N, et al. Elective versus therapeutic neck dissection in node-negative oral cancer. N Engl J Med. 2015; 373: 521–9.
8. Hutchison IL, Ridout F, Cheung SMY, et al. Nationwide randomised trial evaluating elective neck dissection for early stage oral cancer (SEND study) with meta-analysis and concurrent real-world cohort. Br J Cancer. 2019; 121: 827–36.

CHAPTER 11

Elective versus Therapeutic Neck Dissection in Node-Negative Oral Cancer

D'Cruz AK, Vaish R, Kapre N, et al. N Engl J Med. 2015; 373: 521–9.

Reviewed by David A Mitchell

Research Question/Objective

The authors previously described an apparent controversy over whether or not patients with early-stage oral cancers should be treated with elective neck dissection at the time of primary surgery or with therapeutic neck dissection after nodal relapse.[1]

Study Design

A prospective, single-centre randomised controlled clinical trial of patients undergoing surgical treatment of lateralised T stage 1 and 2, N stage 0, oral squamous cell carcinoma (OSCC). Primary site treatment was by transoral excision without reconstruction, and patients were randomly allocated to either ipsilateral neck dissection or watchful waiting followed by neck dissection in the event of nodal relapse. Primary and secondary endpoints were overall survival and disease-free survival.

Sample Size

A total of 596 patients were enrolled between 2004 and 2014 with a median follow-up of 39 months. The paper describes the results for the first 500 recruited patients, as the trial was stopped early on the basis that interim analysis concluded it would no longer be ethically acceptable to recruit into the watchful waiting group.

Follow-Up

As indicated, follow-up was originally planned at 5 years but the trial was stopped early, with a median follow-up of 39 months.

Inclusion/Exclusion Criteria

Consenting adults aged between 18 and 75 years of age with histopathologically proven invasive SCC of the tongue, floor of mouth, or buccal mucosa that met the Union for International Cancer Control (UICC) criteria for tumour stage T1 and T2 lateralised to one side. Included patients had received no previous treatment, consented to transoral excision and had no prior history of head and neck cancer. Exclusion criteria were previous surgery in the head and neck region, upper alveolar or palatal cancers, large heterogenous leukoplakia, or diffuse oral submucous fibrosis.

Intervention or Treatment Received

Transoral excision (without reconstruction) of the primary tumour (by a number of different surgeons) and randomised allocation to either ipsilateral neck dissection or watchful waiting.

Results

Over a greater than 10-year period, 1,281 patients were screened and 596 subsequently underwent randomisation. The paper describes the data from the first 500 patients (245 in the elective surgery group and 255 in the therapeutic surgery group) who had completed at least 9 months of follow-up. The median follow-up in this group was 39 months (interquartile range 16–76). The numbers of patients lost to follow-up were similar in the two groups. Two patients in each group were excluded at late stages in the process.

The tongue was the most common site for the primary tumour. In the elective surgery group, 174 patients underwent selective neck dissection and 60 underwent modified radical neck dissection. It is stated that 10 (5 + 5) patients in the elective surgery group did not undergo their assigned surgical treatment because they went elsewhere or due to "nonadherence." This is despite the actual difference between 243 and 234 being 9.

In terms of overall survival, there were 50 deaths (20.6%) in the elective surgery group and 79 (31.2%). The authors submit complex statistical techniques to demonstrate a statistically significant difference between the two groups at 3 years strongly in favour of the group undergoing neck dissection at the time of primary excisional surgery.

In terms of disease-free survival, there were 81 recurrences (33.3%) in the elective surgery group and 146 (57.7%) in the watchful waiting group. This translated to a 69.5% disease-free survival in the group undergoing neck dissection at the time of ablative surgery for the primary tumour and 45.9% for those allocated to watchful waiting.

Subgroup analyses demonstrated the benefit of undergoing ipsilateral neck dissection at the time of primary surgery. This was also seen across all factors affecting survival.

Patterns of recurrence demonstrated that patients with nodal relapse presented with more advanced stage disease. Depth of invasion appeared to predict nodal involvement markedly between 3 mm (5.6%) and 4 mm (16.9%).

Surprisingly "adverse events" were reported as 6.6% in patients in the elective surgery group and only 3.6% in the watchful waiting/therapeutic surgery group. It has to be assumed that this data was harvested at an early stage before the second group developed nodal recurrence and underwent whatever version of therapeutic neck dissection was carried out. No formal quality of life (QoL) data was collected, so this information is of negligible value.

Study Limitations

The authors highlight a few of the study limitations in their discussion. Notably the use of selective neck dissection (terminology and logistics, described later) as a diagnostic tool to indicate adjuvant radiotherapy meant a higher percentage of patients underwent potentially curative treatment as a direct consequence of this and the apparent use of frozen section control at the time of surgery (which changed the operation from a level I–III dissection to a level I–V dissection). No mention is made of the sublevels, notably levels IIa and IIb.

A paragraph is devoted to explaining the difference between the incidence of nodal relapse in the therapeutic surgery group (45.1%) versus the elective surgery group (29.6%), which seems to suggest a difference in their routine histopathological examination of submitted neck dissection specimens.

There is no discussion in the paper about the number and range of experience of the surgeons involved in performing neck dissection, nor what would be understood as contemporary terminology for neck dissection (describing the levels cleared and the vital structures preserved).

In addition, this study confounded its original outcome measures by including a secondary measure, essentially undescribed in the paper, relating to the role of ultrasound scans (USS) in staging and follow-up of patients with oral cancer. Quite correctly, this data is not highlighted in the final paper but speaks volumes as to the method of original staging of neck disease (USS in comparison to magnetic resonance imaging (MRI), in most developed countries). It highlights the curative benefits if initial staging under-staged neck disease which was then corrected (to some degree) in the group undergoing elective neck dissection (despite the admitted issues around accuracy of "routine" histopathological examination of the neck specimens, the presentation of which is completely undescribed).

This group was then given adjuvant radiotherapy. It can be argued that the elective neck dissection was not only offered better treatment but better diagnosis which led to timely optimal treatment compared to a group which were simply left with inadequate radiological staging and a clinical (plus USS follow-up). It is not surprising to me that the trial was stopped early.

Relevant Studies

Since Crile[2] described a radical approach to curative excision of metastatic cancer of the head and neck in 1906, progressive treatment modification based on patterns of disease spread,[3] and minimising morbidity while providing safe oncological outcome[4] and even a reemphasis on basic anatomy[5] has been such that even before this study claimed to start recruiting prospective data, textbooks[6] were published on the range and variety of neck dissections. It is therefore surprising that so little information is given on the precise techniques and those performing them in such an otherwise apparently well planned and thought out prospective study.

It is also unclear whether or how many of these patients provided data that were actually from the self-stated retrospective analysis published by a similar group of authors in 2009[1] some 5 years after they state in this article they started prospective data collection.

In the late 1990s and early 2000s, adequate data existed to allow rational treatment planning for multidisciplinary management of patients with oral cancer. MRI was well established as the main radiological investigation for staging of the primary site and the neck. This paper introduced a serious confounding factor in that a secondary outcome was the efficacy of USS in follow-up. It appears to also have been used in staging.

On basic clinical grounds patients were therefore likely to have been under-staged. Clearly those having whatever form of elective (selective) neck dissection and were given the advantages of both frozen section and "routine" histopathological assessment of harvested nodes (whatever the average number of nodes may have been) were going to be far more accurately staged and offered the benefit of postoperative radiotherapy, known to improve survival.[7]

In contrast to standard maxillofacial practice in the Western world during that period, no reconstruction was offered to patients in this series even for T2 tumours. It is already known that this is a separate factor for improved survival[8] even though the mechanism is not understood.

The authors apparently spent over 10 years screening and selecting patients for inclusion into this study, which suggests rigor; however, during the data collection period, the guidelines of several developed countries would have strongly supported ipsilateral level I–III/IV neck dissection plus or minus reconstruction. By the time it was published, the United Kingdom was struggling to complete the selective elective neck dissection (SEND) trial (addressing a similar issue) and subsequently published in 2019[9] because many clinicians were already convinced of the benefit of selective (often sparing level IIb) lymph node dissection based on multiple audits and personal data collection.

This was already the gold standard amongst maxillofacial surgical oncologists in most developed countries.

The current controversy over a recommendation supported by the UK National Institute for Clinical Excellence (NICE, www.nice.org.uk/guidance) but rejected by several head and neck clinical organisations (British Association of Head and Neck Oncologists [BAHNO] and the German-Swiss-Austrian Group on Maxillofacial Tumours [DOSAK]) to first offer similar patients sentinel lymph node biopsy (SLNB) exists because of this conviction amongst a majority of such clinicians.

Why should every maxillofacial surgeon read this paper? It is superficially appealing as a properly randomised apparently prospective clinical trial—a rarity in the field of surgery and especially maxillofacial surgery. Its main benefit is that in a time where "evidence-based medicine" is a powerful fashion, reading it carefully accidentally forces us to challenge the tyranny of metrics, and the deliberate ignoring of common sense and careful observational data, and it shows that it does not take complex statistics to prove the obvious.[10]

REFERENCES

1. D'Cruz AK, Siddachari RC, Walvekar RR, et al. Elective neck dissection for the management of the N0 neck in early cancer of the oral tongue: need for a randomized controlled trial. Head Neck. 2009; 31: 618–24.
2. Crile G. Excision of cancer of the head and neck with special reference to the plan of dissection based on one hundred and thirty-two operations. J Am Med Assoc. 1906; 4: 1780–86.
3. Shah JP, Anderson PE. Evolving role of modifications in neck dissection for oral squamous carcinoma. Br J Oral Maxillofac Surg. 1995; 33: 3–8.
4. Gluckman JL, Johnson JT. Surgical Management of Neck Metastases. London: Martin Dunitz, 2003.
5. Mizen KD, Mitchell DA. The anatomical variability of omohyoid and its surgical relevance in oropharyngeal cancer. Br J Oral Maxillofac Surg. 2005; 43: 285–8.
6. Gavilan J, Herranz J, De Santo LW, Gavilan C. Functional and Selective Neck Dissection. New York: Thieme, 2002.
7. Kramer S, Gelber RD, Snow JB, et al. Combined radiation therapy and surgery in the management of advanced head and neck cancer: final report of study 73-03 of the radiation therapy oncology group. Head Neck Surg. 1987; 10: 19–30.
8. Mucke T, Wolff K-D, Wagenpfeil S, et al. Immediate microsurgical reconstruction after tumour ablation predicts survival among patients with oral squamous cell carcinoma. Ann Surg Oncol. 2009; 17: 287–295.
9. Hutchison IL, Ridout F, Cheung SMY, et al. Nationwide randomised trial evaluating elective neck dissection for early stage oral cancer (SEND study) with meta-analysis and concurrent real-world cohort. Br J Cancer. 2019; 121: 827–36.
10. Yeh RW, Valsdottir LR, Yeh MW, et al. Parachute use to prevent death and major trauma when jumping from aircraft: randomized controlled trial. Br Med J. 2018; 363: k5094.

CHAPTER 12

Sentinel European Node Trial (SENT): 3-Year Results of Sentinel Node Biopsy in Oral Cancer

Schilling C, Stoeckli SJ, Haerle SK, et al. Eur J Cancer. 2015; 51: 2777–84.

Reviewed by Jacob D'Souza and Raghuram Boyapati

Research Question/Objective

To assess the safety and reliability of sentinel lymph node biopsy (SNB) as a staging investigation with respect to the accuracy of sentinel node detection, disease recurrence and survival in T1/T2 N0 oral squamous cell carcinomas (OSCC).

To date his is the largest multicentre prospective study in the literature. It helped generate NICE guidelines for the management of T1-T2 N0 OSCC, necessitating discussing with the patients the options for elective neck dissection and SNB.[1]

Study Design

European multicentre prospective observational study, approved by European Organisation for Research and Treatment of Cancer (EORTC) (protocol 24021) carried out between October 2005 and October 2010, incorporating 14 centres. The participating units had undertaken at least 10 validated SNB procedures prior to involvement in this study.

Sample Size

A total of 481 cases were initially recruited in the study. Of these, 66 patients were excluded for various reasons, including breach of protocol ($n = 25$), lost to follow-up ($n = 16$), and radiotherapy to close margins ($n = 17$). The final study group therefore comprised 415 patients.

Intervention Received

All 415 patients received Tc-99m Nano colloid injection 3–24 hours before SNB. The dye was injected at four points around the tumour just prior to the lymph node harvest in 39% of patients. Lymph nodes with radiation count more than three times the background activity were considered sentinel nodes (SNs). Of these, those with the largest radiation count were considered primary SNs. The remaining hot and/or blue nodes were considered second or third echelon nodes.

The harvested SNs were sent for histopathological assessment. Elective neck dissection (END) was offered within 3 weeks if the sentinel node biopsy was positive. All patients were monitored for at least 3 years.

Inclusion Criteria

Patients with OSCC with a clinical tumour size 0.15–4 cm and radiological T1-T2 N0 with previously untreated necks were included in the study. Some tumours of the oropharynx region that were readily accessible were also included.

Exclusion Criteria

Patients with potentially altered lymphatic drainage (previous tumours or neck treatments) and those medically unfit for neck dissection if the SNB was pathological were excluded.

Results

In the 415 patients included, at least one SN was identified in 99.5% cases. Positive sentinel nodes were detected in 23% of cases. False-negative rate occurred in 14% of patients who developed isolated cervical metastasis despite negative SNB, meaning sensitivity of SNB was 86%.

Unexpected drainage of the contrast was seen in 12% cases, be it to contralateral or bilateral LNs. Of these, positive SNBs were pathological in 6% cases.

In patients who underwent completion neck dissection for positive SNs, 85% had no further nodes at histopathological examination.

The 3-year survival figures were as follows: overall survival 88%, disease-free survival 92%, and disease-specific survival 94%, respectively.

Discussion

Approximately 4% of the maxillofacial/head and neck units in the United Kingdom currently carry out SLNB for T1-2 N0 oral carcinomas.[2] The rate of occult metastasis for this group of patients is less than 30%. The sensitivity of SLNs ranges from 86% to 97%,[3–9] with false-negative rates between 4 and 14%. Systemic review confirmed the pooled SN detection rate of 98%, sensitivity of 92%, and negative predictive value of 96%.[9] The overall survival of SN-negative patients is significantly better than that of SN-positive patients.[4,5] Patients with occult node disease whether that is micro- or macro-metastases or isolated tumour cells do worse than those with sentinel node evaluated patients.[10] Therefore, a completion neck dissection should be performed irrespective of the size of metastasis.

There have been advances in diagnostic imaging modalities, such as widespread availability of PET-CT scans. The routinely used ultrasound guided fine needle cytology lacks accuracy in detecting occult metastasis.[11] However, SLNB can reliably detect micro-metastatic disease in more than 99% patients.[2,4–6,12]

In the neck specimen in patients with positive SNs, the SN was the only node containing metastasis in 80% patients.[3,12] The removal of a greater number of uninvolved regional cervical lymph nodes did not correlate with disease free survival,[13] which makes a strong case for the role of SNB in this selected group of patients.

Whereas the blue dye moves rapidly downstream to distal lymph, the nano-colloids are more efficiently trapped, leading to superior identification of SNs. Lymphoseek®, a new SN tracer can potentially reduce the false-negative rates to 2.5% by rapidly clearing the injection site while retaining the colloid in the SNs; however, this may be attributed to the surgeon's expertise. Indocyanine green fluorescence for imaging in the localisation of SNs had a false-negative rate up to 50% and is therefore not recommended.[14]

The use of serial step sectioning and immunohistochemistry can reliably detect micro-metastasis and isolated tumour cells with increased sensitivity compared to traditional histopathological evaluation; however, some clinicians argue that hematoxylin and eosin with immunohistochemistry is sufficient with a negative-predictive value of 96% even though serial step sectioning was not performed.[15]

The role of intraoperative frozen section analysis of SNs has been studied. Positive nodes were identified in 71.4% cases allowing for simultaneous completion neck dissection. While this has perceived advantages, a Japanese multicentre phase 2 trials demonstrated a false-negative rate of 9%.[4]

A significant number of the studied population (25% patients, $n = 103$) had tumours located in the floor of the mouth. In this anatomical subsite, the radioactive shine-through can cause masking of nodes that lie close to the primary tumour. This may be minimised by removal of some of the fatty pre-glandular tissue in this region to enable application of the probe.[16] Some clinicians have suggested excision of the tumour prior to node harvest to avoid this shine-through phenomenon. Same-day protocol may be advantageous because fewer non-SNs were sampled in the SENT study.[12]

The shape of the SN was not an indicator for predicting positive node, but there is a tendency towards a spherical shape when positive.[17]

SLNB has less morbidity compared to elective neck dissection[18] and the cost-effectiveness was proven in the evaluation of 100 hypothetical patients comparing the local excision and elective neck dissection with or without free flap versus wide local excision and SNB.[19]

REFERENCES

1. NICE guidance for early stage oral cancers: [Available from https://www.nice.org.uk/guidance/qs146/chapter/Quality-statement-3-developmental-Sentinel-lymph-node-biopsy]
2. Schilling C, Shaw R, McGurk M. Sentinel lymph node biopsy for oral squamous cell carcinoma. Where are we now? Br J Oral Maxillofac Surg. 2017; 55: 757–62.
3. Schilling C, Stoeckli SJ, McGurk M, et al. Sentinel European node trial (SENT): 3-year results of sentinel node biopsy in oral cancer. Eur J Cancer. 2015; 51: 2777–84.
4. Miura K, Hirakawa H, Uemura H, et al. Sentinel node biopsy for oral cancer: a prospective multicenter phase II trial. Auris Nasus Larynx. 2017; 44: 319–26.
5. Den Toom IJ, de Bree R. Sentinel node biopsy for early-stage oral cavity cancer: the VU University Medical Centre experience. Head Neck. 2015; 37: 573–8.
6. Pezier T, Nixon IJ, Gurney B, et al. Sentinal lymph node biopsy for T1/T2 oral cavity squamous cell carcinoma – a prospective case series. Ann Surg Oncol. 2012; 19: 3528–33.
7. Samant S. Sentinel node biopsy as an alternative to elective neck dissection for staging of early oral carcinoma. Head Neck. 2014; 36: 241–6.
8. Riese CG, Karstadt JA, Schramm A, et al. Validity of sentinel node biopsy in early oral and oropharyngeal carcinoma. J Craniomaxillofac Surg. 2018; 46: 1748–52.
9. Yang Y, Zhou J, Wu H. Diagnostic value of sentinel lymph node biopsy for cT1/T2N0 tongue squamous cell carcinoma: a meta-analysis. Eur Arch Otorhinolaryngol. 2017; 274: 3843–52.
10. Broglie MA, Haerle SK, Huber GF, Stoeckli SJ. Occult metastases detected by sentinel node biopsy in patients with early oral and oropharyngeal squamous cell carcinomas: impact on survival. Head Neck. 2013; 35: 660–6.
11. Chaturvedi P, Data S, Arya S, et al. Prospective study of ultrasound-guided fine-needle aspiration cytology and sentinel node biopsy in the staging of clinically negative T1 and T2 oral cancer. Head Neck. 2015; 37: 1504–8
12. Tartaglione G, Rubello D, McGurk M. Sentinel node in Oral cancer: the nuclear medicine aspects. A survey from the sentinel European node trial. Clin Nucl Med. 2016; 41: 534–42.
13. Ampil FL, Caldito G, Ghali GE, Baluna RG. Does the negative node count affect disease-free survival in early-stage oral cavity cancer? J Oral Maxillofac Surg. 2009; 67: 2473–5.
14. Al-Dam A, Heiland M, Assaf AT, et al. Sensitivity and specificity of sentinel lymph node biopsy in patients with oral squamous cell carcinomas using indocyanine green fluorescence imaging. J Craniomaxillofac Surg. 2018; 46: 1379–84.
15. Bell RB, Markiewicz MR, Dierks EJ, Gregoire CE, Rader A. Thin serial step sectioningn of sentinel lymph node biopsy specimen may not be necessary to accurately stage the neck in oral Squamous cell carcinoma. J Oral Maxillofac Surg. 2013; 71: 1268–77.
16. Stoeckli SJ, Huebner T, Huber GF, Broglie MA. Technique for reliable sentinel node biopsy in squamous cell carcinomas of the floor of mouth. Head Neck. 2016; 38: 1367–72.
17. Langhans L, von Buchwald C. Evaluations of sentinel lymph node size and shape as a predictor of occult metastasis in patients with squamous cell carcinoma of the oral cavity. Eur Arch Otorhinolaryngol. 2013; 270: 249–54.
18. Murer K, Huber GF, Haile SR, Stoeckli SJ. Comparison of morbidity between sentinel node biopsy and elective neck dissection for treatment of the N0 neck in patients with oral squamous cell carcinoma. Head Neck. 2011; 33: 1260–4.
19. O'Connor R, Pezier T, Schilling C, McGurk M. The relative cost of sentinel lymph node biopsy in early oral cancer. J Craniomaxillofac Surg. 2013; 41: 721–7.

CHAPTER 13

A Study of Facial Growth in Patients with Unilateral Cleft Lip and Palate Treated by the Oslo CLP Team

Semb G. Cleft Palate Craniofac J. 1991; 28: 1–21.

Reviewed by Alistair G Smyth

Research Question/Objective

Facial growth in children with cleft lip and palate is an important outcome measure. This study was undertaken to assess craniofacial development of patients with repaired unilateral cleft lip and palate (UCLP) treated by the CLP Team in Oslo and compare with published data. Factors including cleft subtype, gender, and surgical variables were also analysed for their potential impact on facial growth.

Study Design

A retrospective, single-centre longitudinal survey over a 25-year period (1954–1979). Facial growth was assessed from serial lateral and frontal cephalometric radiographs.

Sample Size

A total of 257 children were included.

Follow-up

According to the Oslo team protocol, serial cephalometric radiographs were obtained during growth; in many cases up to early adult life.

Inclusion/Exclusion Criteria

Children born between 1954 and 1979 were included and treated only within the Oslo CLP Team for complete UCLP, and who had a minimum of two pairs of lateral and frontal cephalograms taken at least 1 year apart. Patients were excluded if they only had one pair of cephalograms, if there was a history of other malformation, or learning difficulties. Five patients underwent jaw osteotomies in their late teens and were also excluded.

Treatment Received

No patients within the study received either presurgical orthopaedics or orthodontic treatment in the deciduous dentition. All patients underwent staged primary repair with initial lip and anterior palate repair with a superiorly based single layer vomer flap in infancy and subsequent posterior cleft palate repair in early childhood. No palatal releasing incisions were made at the time of the first stage of surgery which included vomer flap. From 1953 a Le Mesurier lip repair was performed, but in 1961 a Millard repair was introduced. The timing of the lip repair from 1953 was 6 months of age; however, this reduced to 3 months of age from 1968 onwards.

The subsequent repair of the remaining posterior cleft palate was carried out using a von Langenbeck repair in all patients. Lateral palatal release incisions were therefore performed in all patients, a muscle dissection was included, and the pterygoid hamuli were routinely in-fractured. The posterior cleft palate repair was initially undertaken at 3–4 years, but this gradually reduced during the study period and by 1974 all palate repairs were completed by 18 months of age. Bone grafting of the alveolar cleft was introduced in 1977 and carried out on patients between 8 and 11 years of age. Secondary cleft lip and nose revision was carried out in almost all patients, usually after completion of orthodontics (around 15 years of age). When required, surgery for velopharyngeal insufficiency was carried out preferably before the child started school (7 years of age) using a superiorly based pharyngeal flap.

Cephalometric radiographic records of patients with UCLP were collected by the cleft team orthodontist. From 1973 this included annual cephalometric records (frontal and lateral) under standardised conditions, for the majority of patients with complete clefts from 5 years of age.

The cephalograms were digitised using standardised bony and soft tissue landmarks and reference planes. All radiographs were digitised twice at the same sitting by the author who was the head of the dental unit attached to the Oslo CLP Team. Forty-five bony skeletal variables (23 angular and 22 linear) and 27 soft tissue variables (13 angular and 14 linear) were calculated from the lateral cephalograms. Six variables were also measured from the frontal anteroposterior cephalograms. The lateral and frontal radiographs from 30 randomly selected patients were digitised twice by the author one week apart to assess reliability. Mean values of cephalometric variables from this cohort of UCLP patients were compared to known standard values from a non-cleft population (Bolton standards).

Results

A total of 257 children with UCLP treated over the 25-year period were included (176 males; 81 females). Of these, 177 were left-sided and 80 right-sided (2:1). Of the 257, 80 (31%) included a Simonart's band. Thirty-six patients (10.1%) had a Le Mesurier lip repair with vomer flap, and the remaining 221 patients had a Millard repair with vomer flap. All patients had a von Langenbeck repair of the posterior palate. One hundred and sixty-eight patients (65.4%) received an alveolar bone graft. Sixty-nine patients (27%) underwent secondary surgery for closure of symptomatic fistula and 52 (20%) underwent pharyngeal flap surgery. Twenty-two surgeons were involved in the surgery over the 25-year period. The data from 28 variables is presented in table form showing the mean value and standard deviation separately for males and females at yearly intervals from age 5 or younger to age 18 or older.

The skeletal and soft tissue features were characterised by a short and retrusive maxilla, vertical elongation of the anterior face, and a retrusive mandible. Posterior face height was reduced and cranial base angulation was slightly increased, as was interocular distance. The pattern of growth differed from non-cleft individuals, with almost no increase in length of the maxilla between 5 and 18 years of age. A marked and progressive reduction in maxillary prominence (S-N-SS) of 5.4 degrees was observed in the pooled UCLP patients which compares with an expected increase of 3.3 degrees in the non-cleft data. Mandibular retrusion was observed in the sample with an increase of only 3.8 degrees in mandibular prominence (S-N-PG), when compared with the 6.2 degree increase from pooled Bolton standards. The facial soft tissue profile differed from non-cleft individuals with nasal growth in a more backward and downward direction, a receded upper lip, and a progressively straighter profile. Further analysis of the surgical effects on facial growth failed to reveal any differences between the surgical groups and surgical variation during the 25-year period. The cephalometric outcomes are compared with outcomes from other centres and were found to be similar. Shortcomings of the previous reports in the literature in addition to those within the present study are acknowledged.

Effect of Surgical Variation

These included changes in technique for lip repair, timing of primary surgery, number of surgeons involved, and the variable provision of secondary surgery. Although surgery was performed according to the protocol at the time, senior surgeons would often carry out the primary lip and anterior palate repair, while junior surgeons would participate in the repair of the posterior cleft palate. It is suggested that despite these variations, pooling of the subjects born over the 25-year period remains valid and that independent analysis of surgical effects failed to reveal any differences within the surgical subgroups.

Comparison with Other Reports

Growth outcomes are similar to those in other publications for Caucasian children treated for the same condition. Direct comparisons are difficult due to differences in cephalometric landmarks, analyses and variations in sample size, age, and cleft subtypes.

Influence of a Vomer Flap on Facial Growth

The paper suggests that the vomer flap independently may not be detrimental to facial growth. This is based on the observation that the outcomes for maxillary prominence (S-N-SS) and upper face angulation (NSL-NL) in this and other centres who carried out the same protocol[1-3], did not differ from other centres who performed delayed hard palate closure between 4 and 8 years of age.[4-6] It is also postulated that hard palate repair at 4–8 years of age could still have an adverse effect on maxillary development and that it is only when hard palate repair is exceptionally delayed, as in the Marburg sample when the mean age at repair was 13.2 years, that a beneficial effect on maxillary growth is apparent. This benefit is arguably outweighed by the impaired speech outcome associated with the delay in palate repair.[7]

Study Limitations

The author acknowledged several limitations of the study including the evolving protocol over the 25-year period, the numerous surgeons involved, and the potential impact of secondary surgery. Nonetheless, constants over the 25-year period in all patients were vomer flap repair of the hard palate at the same time as lip repair and the subsequent von Langenbeck repair of the posterior palate. The number of patients excluded (inadequate records, other malformation, or learning difficulty) is not provided. The cephalometric assessments were performed only by the author from the team.

Relevant Studies

Although the advantages of a vomer flap are highlighted (early separation of the nasal and oral cavities, low rate of symptomatic fistula, acceptable arch form, and good foundation for mixed dentition alveolar bone grafting) some authors have criticised its use during cleft palate repair, suggesting that scarring at the premaxillary-vomerine suture may inhibit future mid facial growth.[8] Friede and Johanson reported poor facial growth in their cohort of patients treated with a three-stage surgical protocol including vomer flap.[9] However, the posterior cleft palate repair was completed using a "push back" technique which was likely to impact facial growth.

The Scandcleft randomised trials, which started in 1997. included three different surgical procedures, one of which was the "Oslo" protocol of vomer flap closure of the hard palate at the same time as lip repair at 3–4 months, followed by closure of the remaining posterior cleft palate at 12 months. However, results from the trial did not provide any statistical evidence that one technique provided any better facial growth than the others, assessed by dental arch relationship at 5 years of age.[10] As in this Semb study, it is possible that despite the initial use of a vomer flap, the major iatrogenic impact on facial growth resulted from the subsequent posterior cleft palate repair, particularly if that includes a von Langenbeck repair, requiring lateral palatal incisions, wide undermining of the palatal fibromucosa, and in-fracture of the pterygoid hamuli. Sommerlad reported that in 48 patients (between 1993 and 1997) with complete unilateral cleft lip and palate where the treatment included a vomerine flap, lateral incisions/oral flaps were avoided in 44 cases (92%) (chapter 14).[11] While this may not be achievable in all cases of UCLP managed with a vomer flap, nonetheless it would be preferable to repair the posterior cleft palate without need for lateral incisions/oral flaps when reasonable to do so, with the intention of reducing palatal scarring to facilitate better facial growth.

REFERENCES

1. Enemark H, Bolund S, Jorgensen I, et al. Evaluation of unilateral cleft lip and palate treatment: long term results. Cleft Palate J. 1990; 27: 354–61.
2. Rygh P, Sirinavin I. Craniofacial morphology in six-year-old Norwegian boys with complete cleft of the lip and palate. Swed Dent J Suppl. 1982; 15: 203–13.
3. Dahl E. Craniofacial morphology in congenital clefts of the lip and palate. An x-ray cephalometric study of young adult males. Thesis. Acta Odontol Scand. 1970; 28: Suppl 57.
4. Hotz M, Gnoinski W. Comprehensive care of cleft lip and palate children at Zürich University: a preliminary report. Am J Orthod. 1976; 70: 481–504.
5. Smahel Z, Mullerova Z. Effects of primary periosteoplasty on facial growth in unilateral cleft lip and palate: 10 year follow-up. Cleft Palate J. 1988; 25: 356–61.
6. Friede H, Moller M, Lilja J, et al. Facial morphology and occlusion at the stage of early mixed dentition in cleft lip and palate patients treated with delayed closure of the hard palate. Scand J Plast Reconstr Surg. 1987; 21: 65–71.
7. Bardach J, Morris HL, Olin WH, et al. Late results of primary veloplasty: the Marburg project. Plast Reconstr Surg. 1984; 73: 207–17.
8. Delaire J, Precious D. Avoidance of the use of vomerine mucosa in primary surgical management of velopalatine clefts. Oral Surg Oral Med Oral Pathol. 1985; 60: 589–97.
9. Friede H, Johanson B. A follow-up study of cleft children treated with vomer flap as part of a three-stage soft tissue surgical procedure. Facial morphology and dental occlusion. Scand J Plast Reconstr Surg. 1977; 11: 45–57.
10. Heliovaara A, Kuseler A, Skaare P, et al. Scandcleft randomised trials of primary surgery for unilateral cleft lip and palate: 6. Dental arch relationships in 5-year-olds. J Plast Surg Hand Surg. 2017; 51: 52–57.
11. Sommerlad B. A technique for cleft palate repair. Plast Reconstr Surg. 2003; 112: 1542–8.

CHAPTER 14

A Technique for Cleft Palate Repair

Sommerlad BC. Plast Reconstr Surg. 2003; 112: 1542–8.

Reviewed by Tom WM Walker and Alistair RM Cobb

Research Question/Objective

Primary

To assess the outcome of intravelar veloplasty palatal repair as measured by number of patients requiring secondary velopharyngeal surgery within 10 years of cleft repair (patients operated on between 1978 and 1992).

The outcome was also examined in successive 5-year periods within this 15-year timeframe.

Secondary

To identify the number of patients requiring von Langenbeck lateral releasing incisions (1993–1997 patients).

To identify the effect of the vomerine flap on the need for von Langenbeck lateral releasing incisions (1993–1997 patients).

To identify the fistula repair rate (1993–1997 patients).

Study Design

This is a large retrospective case series with a primary outcome measure of rate of secondary velopharyngeal surgery within 10 years of cleft repair.

Sample Size

The study included 442 children who had primary palate repair between 1978 and 1992 inclusive.

88 repairs were performed between 1978 and 1982, 162 between 1983 and 1987, and 192 between 1988 and 1992.

It also examined 285 children who had repairs between 1993 and 1997.

Follow-up

All patients had at least 10-year follow-up.

Patients operated on between 1978 and 1987 had up to 25-year follow-up. Some patients in the 1988–1992 cohort had up to 15-year follow-up.

Inclusion/Exclusion Criteria

Children with Cleft palate (CP), unilateral cleft lip and palate (UCLP), bilateral cleft lip and palate (BCLP) treated by a single surgeon with a 10-year follow-up.

Surgery was normally at 6 months old, but all before 12 months.

No exclusions (for example syndromic patients).

Intervention or Treatment Received

Patients were treated with an intra velar veloplasty by a single operator. Using a marginal incision, the nasal and oral mucosa were dissected from the palatal musculature and the three layers closed separately with the latter realigned with a more normal anatomical relationship.

This more radical dissection and retro-positioning of the tissues was argued to be better for palatal function when compared to more traditional release techniques.

Results

The secondary velopharyngeal surgery rate decreased from 10.2% to 4.9% to 4.6% in successive 5-year periods within this 15 study year period.

Amongst patients with UCLP, 80% did not require von Langenbeck releasing incisions. This was 92% if a vomerine flap had been used.

In CP patients, 84% did not require von Langenbeck releasing incisions. This ranged from 59% in complete clefts of the palate to 100% in isolated clefts of the soft palate.

In patients with BCLP, 29% did not require von Langenbeck releasing incisions.

The fistula repair rate was 14% in UCLP, 35% in BCLP, and 12% in clefts of the secondary palate. The overall fistula repair rate was 15% and 12% if BCLP patients were excluded.

The results showed that it took procedures on 88 patients to be able to reduce the rate of secondary velopharyngeal surgery from 10.2% to 4.9%.

Study Limitations

The paper reports that in 1991 the surgeon changed the technique by using an operative microscope. There is no mention of objective assessment on the indication for secondary velopharyngeal surgery and the need for follow-up surgery is a broad surrogate marker for velopharyngeal insufficiency (VPI).

Relevant Studies

Historically cleft palate repair was primarily aimed at the separation of the oral and nasal cavities and an attempt to lengthen the soft palate, which did not take into account the abnormal muscular anatomy of the soft palate. Failure to accurately correct the anatomy restricts the potential for normal physiological function and can result in poor speech and velopharyngeal incompetence.

Sommerlad[1] sought to reconstruct the patho-anatomy first described by Fergusson in 1844 and improve on the technique described by Kriens[2] and Cutting et al.[3] This has been done by the effect of multiple small gains with a precise and careful technique and a consideration of the effect of every surgical step taken. The use of saline to wash off blood rather than swabs, topical adrenaline rather than diathermy, minimisation of dissection, and a use of a vomerine flap to reduce the need for lateral relieving incisions have all helped to reduce the need for further speech surgery and yield good results in terms of speech and palate function.

Similar results have also been achieved by Cutting et al.,[3] who identified a secondary surgical intervention rate of 6.3% and Andrades et al.,[4] who demonstrated a reduction in secondary surgery for VPI from 29% to 6.7% after introduction of the Sommerlad palate repair.

The true value of the technique is judged by the effect it has on cleft speech outcomes.

The technique has also been used by Sommerlad in the re-repair of palates— instead of pharyngeal flaps or pharyngoplasty. There are well recognised and significant early and late morbidity and indeed mortality with pharyngeal surgery for VPI. Sommerlad suggests that a palate re-repair is more physiological. It aims to improve the function and length of the soft palate and does not distort the anatomy of the pharynx and rely on the creation of a permanent obstruction in the pharynx to achieve velopharyngeal competence.

In a detailed study of 85 patients with a mean age of 10.8 years (range 3.2–48.8), Sommerlad and Mehendale[5] analysed the effect of the microscope assisted intravelar veloplasty (IVVP) on velar morhphology, function, and speech outcomes in consecutive patients. Seventy percent of the patients had already had an IVVP undertaken as part of their primary repair.

There were significant improvements in hyper-nasality, intelligibility, nasal emission, and nasal turbulence. Significant improvements were identified in velar function also. There were no cases of early postoperative or secondary haemorrhage. There were no recorded cases of sleep apnea or obstructive nasal symptoms. Ten patients (11.8%) required further velopharyngeal surgery, however, it was possible to perform a less obstructive pharyngoplasty than would otherwise have been necessary. Although ten patients required a second procedure that could have been carried out at the same time as the re-repair—75 patients avoided having pharyngeal surgery that can tether the velum and cause obstructive symptoms.

The use of a microscope allows more radical dissection and retro-positioning of the muscles. Indeed, 84% had some form of previous IVVP undertaken, and a more radical approach in the re-repair resulted in a decrease in the speech characteristics associated with VPI. The authors suggest that the reason for this may be that previous IVVP were not as radical as they could have been.

Comparison is made with Furlow veloplasty,[6] as this has been used to treat secondary VPI because it lengthens the velum and repositions the muscle. It is argued that the Furlow repair does not increase the functional length of the palate, and asymmetrical VP closure has been noted.[7]

IVVP aims to reconstruct the palate anatomically and allow it to function as physiologically as possible. Careful and precise surgical dissection with microscopic assistance has led to improved results in speech outcomes and fewer patients requiring additional procedures for their speech. It also appears to be useful in the re-repair of the palate. It is a procedure that takes time to master—and therefore it may not be used as much in North America where cleft is not managed in the same high-volume organized networks as in the United Kingdom, despite increasing evidence as to the benefits of being treated in high-volume centres.[8]

REFERENCES

1. Sommerlad BC. A technique for cleft palate repair. Plast Reconstr Surg. 2003; 112: 1542–8.
2. Kriens OB. An anatomical approach to veloplasty. Plast Reconstr Surg. 1969; 43: 29–41.
3. Cutting C, Rosenbaum J, Rovati L. The technique of muscle repair in the cleft soft palate. Oper Tech Plast Reconstr Surg. 1995; 2: 215–22.
4. Andrades P, Espinosa-de-los-Monteros A, Shell DH IV, et al. The importance of radical intravelar veloplasty during two- flap palatoplasty. Plast Reconstr Surg. 2008; 122: 1121–30.
5. Sommerlad BC, Mehendale FV, Birch MJ, et al. Palate re-repair revisited. Cleft Palate Craniofac J. 2002; 39: 295–307.

6. Chen PK, Wu JT, Chen YR, Noordhoff MS. Correction of secondary velopharyngeal insufficiency in cleft palate patients with the Furlow palatoplasty. Plastic Reconstr Surg. 1994; 94: 933–41.
7. Chen PK, Wu J, Hung KF, Chen YR, Noordhoof MS. Surgical correction of submucous cleft palate with Furlow palatoplasty. Plast Reconstr Surg. 1996; 97: 1136–46.
8. Wes AM, Mazzaferano D, Naran S, Bartlett SP, Taylor JA. Cleft palate repair: does hospital case-volume impact outcomes or cost? Plas Recon Surg. 2018; 141: 1193–200.

CHAPTER 15

Bilateral Cleft Lip and Nose Repair: Review

Penfold C, Dominguez-Gonzalez S. Br J Oral Maxillofac Surg. 2011; 49: 165–71.

Reviewed by Anusha Hennedige and Victoria Beale

Objective

Discussion on recent trends and controversies in primary cheilorhinoplasty for bilateral cleft lip and palate (BCLP).

Study Focus

The paper focuses on five areas of controversy in bilateral cleft lip and nose repair:

1. Timing and staging of repair
2. Use of presurgical orthopaedics
3. Reconstruction of the philtrum and midline vermilion
4. Reconstruction of nasolabial muscles
5. Correction of nasal deformity

Outcome of Discussion

1. **Timing and staging of repair:** This can be a one- or two-stage repair.[1] In one-stage repair, obtaining satisfactory reconstruction of the muscle across the defect, with a protuberant premaxilla, can be a challenge. The two-stage repair can be approached by initial bilateral lip adhesions, which acts as a form of presurgical orthopaedics and helps control the protrusive maxilla. However, there is no evidence that it improves long-term outcomes. The one-side first approach facilitates staged closure of the alveolar clefts with vomer flaps. The disadvantage here is that at second-stage repair, the remaining unilateral cleft can be difficult to close if the premaxilla has rotated to the repaired side. The one-stage repair is the preferred method for repair of BCLP.

2. **Use of presurgical orthopaedics:** The main objective is to retro-position the maxilla and enable a tension-free repair of the lip.[2] However, there is no evidence that it improves outcomes.[3-5] Nasoalveolar moulding (NAM) aims to reshape the nasal tip by lengthening the columella and

repositioning the maxilla.[6] It shows promising results, but long-term outcome has yet to be formally reported. It is technically challenging and time-consuming and requires a high degree of parental cooperation. It also does not correct the increased alar base width or nasolabial angle.

3. **Reconstruction of the philtrum and midline vermilion:** The Manchester-type repair results in a midline segment of vermilion that looks abnormal and a "whistle deformity" as muscles are not reconstructed across the prolabium. Mulliken advocates thinning the width of the prolabium with a distance of 3.5–4 mm between the peaks of the cupid's bow and decreasing to 2 mm at the columellar-labial junction.[7,8] Brusati advocates conserving a small triangle of prolabial vermilion in cases where there is little white roll in the lateral segment.[9] In addition, wet prolabial mucosa can be used to augment the premaxillary lining of the fornix or incorporated in the anterior sulcus wall.

4. **Reconstruction of nasolabial muscles:** There is little agreement in the literature about the method of reconstruction of nasolabial muscles. Many authors advocate reconstruction of the superior oblique component of the orbicularis oris muscle either to the anterior nasal spine or to the base of the nasal septum, which restores continuity of the middle muscle ring. Delaire emphasised the importance of reconstructing the upper nasolabial muscle ring by suturing the transverse nasalis muscle to the anterior nasal spine, which produces a functional lip that can pout and will lengthen over time.[10]

5. **Correction of nasal deformity:** The junction of the columella and lip should be established at a point midway between the prolabial mucocutaneous junction and the planned superior internal angle of the nostril. This anticipates a spontaneous increase in lip height and complements retrieval of the columella from inside the nose. Primary surgical reshaping of the alar cartilages has been advocated by several surgeons via intranasal incisions and the reshaped lower alar cartilages supported by direct suturing or long-term nasal splints.[8,11,12]

There are three main themes to correction of nasal deformity: (1) conservative with no extra incisions; (2) retrograde technique and (3) anterograde technique. In the conservative technique, the alar cartilages are approached medially from the prolabium by tunnelling under the columella and laterally from the alar bases. This is combined with a limited amount of subperichondrial nasal septal dissection for repositioning of the medial crura.

In the retrograde technique, the approach is posterior to the medial crura and utilises an extended prolabial incision up through the membranous septum. The alar cartilages are hence accessed via a retrograde approach.

Lastly, the anterograde approach is anterior to the medial crura where the prolabial incision is continued subcutaneously up the lateral aspect of the columella superficial to the alar cartilages, together with a separate intranasal rim incision. Although this increases columella length, it also increases nasolabial angle, columellar, and inter-alar width, which are unsatisfactory results.

Primary rhinoplasty with reshaping of the alar cartilage and direct suturing produces early satisfactory results, but these are not always predictable.[11]

REFERENCES

1. Ross RB, MacNamera MC. Effect of presurgical infant orthopedics on facial esthetics in complete bilateral cleft lip and palate. Cleft Palate Craniofac J. 1994; 31: 68–73.
2. Peat JH. Effects of presurgical oral orthopedics on bilateral complete clefts of the lip and palate. Cleft Palate J. 1982; 19: 100–3.
3. Robertson N, Shaw W, Volp C. The changes produced by presurgical orthopedic treatment of bilateral cleft lip and palate. Plast Reconstr Surg. 1977; 59: 87–93.
4. Berkowitz S, Mejia M, Bystrik A. A comparison of the effects of the Latham–Millard procedure with those of a conservative treatment approach for dental occlusion and facial aesthetics in unilateral and bilateral complete cleft lip and palate: Part I. Dental occlusion. Plast Reconstr Surg. 2004; 113: 1–18.
5. Randall P. A lip adhesion operation in cleft lip surgery. Plast Reconstr Surg. 1965; 35: 371–6.
6. Mulliken JB. Bilateral cleft lip. Clin Plast Surg. 2004; 31: 209–20.
7. Mulliken JB, Wu JK, Padwa BL. Repair of bilateral cleft lip: review, revisions, and reflections. J Craniofac Surg. 2003; 14: 609–20.
8. Delaire J. Fentes labiales congénitales. In Lévignac J (Ed.): Chirugie des lèvres. Paris: Masson, 1991.
9. Brusati R, Mannucci N, Mommaerts MY. The Delaire philosophy of cleft lip and palate repair. In Ward Booth P, Schendel SA, Hausamen JE (Eds.): Maxillofacial Surgery. London: Churchill Livingstone, 2006.
10. Broadbent TR, Woolf RM. Cleft lip nasal deformity. Ann Plast Surg. 1984; 12: 216–34.
11. Talmant JC. Cleft rhinoplasty. In Ward Booth P, Schendel SA, Hausamen JE (Eds.): Maxillofacial Surgery, 1st ed. London: Churchill Livingstone, 1999.
12. Trott JA, Mohan N. A preliminary report on open tip rhinoplasty at the time of lip repair in unilateral cleft lip and palate: the Alor Setar experience. Br J Plast Surg. 1993; 46: 363–70.

CHAPTER **16**

Cleft Lip, Cleft Palate, and Velopharyngeal Insufficiency

Fisher DM, Sommerlad BC. Plast Reconstr Surg. 2011; 128: 342e–60e.

Reviewed by Simon van Eeden

This paper starts with the learning objectives and a summary, which provides a useful introduction and sets the tone for the paper. After reading this article, the participant should be able to:

1. Recognise the clinical features associated with unilateral cleft lip, bilateral cleft lip, the cleft lip nasal deformity, cleft palate and velopharyngeal insufficiency (VPI).
2. Describe the most frequently used techniques for repair of cleft lip and palate.
3. Diagnose and treat VPI.

Summary

This article provides an introduction to the anatomical and clinical features of the primary deformities associated with unilateral cleft lip–cleft palate, bilateral cleft lip–cleft palate, and cleft palate. The diagnosis and management of secondary velopharyngeal insufficiency (VPI) are discussed. The accompanying videos demonstrate the features of the cleft lip nasal deformities and reliable surgical techniques for unilateral cleft lip repair, bilateral cleft lip repair, and radical intravelar veloplasty (IVVP).

Study Design

A continuing medical education article which includes:

- Good anatomical description of unilateral and bilateral cleft lips, cleft nasal deformity, and cleft palates.
- Outline of bone grafting philosophy with a clear explanation of why the authors prefer secondary bone grafting to gingivoperioplasty (GPP).
- Principles of unilateral lip repair are concisely explained with reference to and explanation of different repairs and their advantages and shortfalls. The article provides detail about the rotation-advancement technique popularised by Millard[1,2] by firstly describing the technique

and then outlining the advantages and disadvantages. This is followed by a brief summary of modifications to the rotation advancement technique described by Millard to address its disadvantages and a description of the Chang-Gung modifications publicised by Mohler[3] and Noordhof.[4] Fisher then describes his technique and the underlying rationale for this.[5] A short paragraph on the adoption of a hybrid technique follows, the preferred option for Sommerlad, which brings together the best features of several techniques.

- Basic principles of bilateral cleft lip are outlined and relevant references provided. Videos of the lip markings can be accessed from the article. The basic principles followed in the referenced articles are summarised.[6–9]
- Some of the common protocols for closure of the palate in cases where the cleft involves the lip and alveolus are described and their references also provided.
- Techniques for closure of the hard palate are discussed and described in some detail, including the Von Langenbeck technique,[10] the Veau-Wardill-Kilner pushback technique and its disadvantages[11–15] and the two-flap technique and its modifications.[16,17] The authors disagree on their approach for this. Fisher is more liberal in his use of relieving incisions to minimise fistula formation,[18] while Sommerlad uses relaxing incisions in less than 10% of cases with a slightly higher fistula rate (chapter 14).[19] Sommerlad uses a superiorly based vomerine flap to close the hard palate in unilateral cleft lip and palate (UCLP) cases.[19]
- Soft palate closure focuses on the importance of the palatal musculature with emphasis on the radical muscle repositioning technique described by Sommerlad.[20,21] There is also access to videos of this technique through the article. A brief description of the popular Furlow technique follows with readers being referred to the original articles.[22,23] Disadvantages of the Furlow technique are also mentioned and ways in which to minimise these by following the Children's Hospital of Pennsylvania modification are described and referenced.[24]

A brief explanation of the diagnosis and management of VPI follows. The special investigations used to aid the diagnosis and treatment of VPI, namely nasoendoscopy (NE) and lateral videofluoroscopy (LV), are explained. The two authors have differing philosophies for the management of VPI: Fisher uses NE to aid treatment decisions and will use a Furlow technique for small VP gaps and a high closure rating, a sphincter pharyngoplasty for those cases of poor lateral wall movement and a midline pharyngeal flap for those with non-coronal closure pattern and low closure ratings. The different patterns of velopharyngeal closure are described in this article. See Figure 16.1. Fischer references the publication on his work to provide evidence for his decision-making and philosophy.[25]

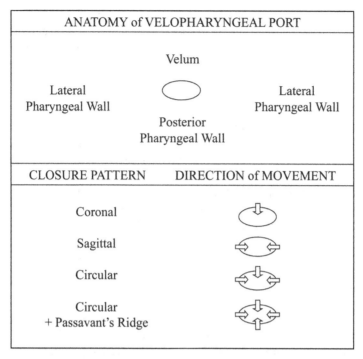

Figure 16.1   Patterns of velopharyngeal closure. (Adapted from Skolnick ML, McCall GN, Barnes M. The sphincteric mechanism of velopharyngeal closure. Cleft Palate J. 1973; 10: 286–305.)

Sommerlad on the other hand will predominantly use LV to inform his treatment decisions and will reposition the palatal muscles more posteriorly in those cases where the muscles appear anterior on the LV. Similar success rates using this approach are referred to in the article.[26,27] In those cases where the palatal re-repair has not adequately corrected the VPI, a posterior pharyngeal wall augmentation (modified Hynes) pharyngoplasty is carried out.[28,29]

• Correction of the cleft nasal deformity (rhinoplasty) is briefly alluded to in this article. Opportunities to carry out nasal correction during the patient's treatment journey are itemised and minimising iatrogenic damage to the nasal skin and the underlying skeleton is emphasised.

Relevant Studies

Several papers that are either referenced by the authors or have been published since on this article are also worth reading and are detailed in the following paragraphs.

Fisher[5] described the background and philosophy behind his cleft lip repair technique and went through the lip markings for the repair in great anatomical detail, explaining the adjustments necessary in the technique to achieve a balanced symmetrical lip in his own article in *Plastic and Reconstructive Surgery* in 2005.

Sommerlad first described the use of the operating microscope for cleft palate repair and pharyngoplasty and the advantages in doing so in 2003.[30] The use of the operating microscope by Sommerlad underpins his technique for cleft palate repair, which is described in a detailed stepwise fashion in a second paper (Chapter 14).[19] The speech and fistula results following this repair are also published in this paper. The speech outcomes, which are excellent in the round, are also shown to improve with operative experience. Sommerlad therefore provides strong evidence for the use of this technique to repair clefts of the palate.

Becker and Hansson demonstrated improved fistula rates of 5% using the Sommerlad IVVP technique, which they attribute to the liberal use of Von Langenbeck relieving incisions.[31]

Moar et al. also reported on the fistula rate following Sommerlad repair across six units in the United Kingdom.[32] While the rate of relieving incisions was higher in this study compared to the original Sommerlad paper, the incidence of fistula rate was very similar. There were also more fistulae in those patients who had relieving incisions (may relate to wider clefts) and in those with bilateral clefts of the lip and palate, which differs from the results in the Becker study.[31]

Sommerlad presented his results of radical muscle repositioning to address velopharyngeal incompetence in a series of articles, demonstrating the use of this technique to measurably improve velar function and speech without the disadvantages of nasopharyngeal obstruction prevalent in flap techniques used to address velopharyngeal incompetence.[27,28]

In a systematic review, Téblick et al. evaluated the influence of cleft palate closure technique on middle ear function and speech.[33] The Sommerlad and Furlow techniques were found to have better hearing and speech outcomes compared to other techniques used for cleft palate closure.

REFERENCES

1. Millard DR Jr. Complete unilateral clefts of the lip. Plast Reconstr Surg. 1960; 25: 595–605.
2. Millard DR. Extensions of the rotation-advancement principle for wide unilateral cleft lips. Plast Reconstr Surg. 1968; 42: 535–44.
3. Mohler LR. Unilateral cleft lip repair. Plast Reconstr Surg. 1987; 80: 511–7.
4. Noordhoff MS. The Surgical Technique for the Unilateral Cleft Lip-Nasal Deformity. Taipei, Taiwan: Noordhoff Craniofacial Foundation, 1997.

5. Fisher DM. Unilateral cleft lip repair: an anatomical subunit approximation technique. Plast Reconstr Surg. 2005; 116: 61–71.
6. Mulliken JB. Principles and techniques of bilateral complete cleft lip repair. Plast Reconstr Surg. 1985; 75: 477–87.
7. Mulliken JB. Primary repair of bilateral complete cleft lip and nasal deformity. Plast Reconstr Surg. 2001; 108: 181–94.
8. Chen PKT, Noordhoff MS. Bilateral cleft lip and nose repair. In Losee JE, Kirschner RE (Eds.): Comprehensive Cleft Care. New York: McGraw-Hill, 2009.
9. Fisher DM. Bilateral cleft lip. In Guyuron B, Eriksson E, Persing J (Eds.): Plastic Surgery. Philadelphia: Saunders, 2009.
10. von Langenbeck B. Weitere Erfahrungen im Gebiete der Uranoplastik mittels Ablosung des mucosperiostalen Gaumenuberzuges. Arch Klin Chir. 1864; 5: 1–70.
11. Veau V. Division Palatine. Paris: Masson, 1931.
12. Veau V, Ruppie C. Anatomie chirurgicale de la division palatine: considerations operatoires. Rev Chir. 1922; 20: 1–30.
13. Wardill WEM. Technique of operation for cleft lip and palate. Br J Surg. 1937; 25: 117–30.
14. Kilner TP. Cleft lip and palate repair technique. In Maingot R (Ed.): Postgraduate Surgery. Vol. 3. London: Medical Publishers, 1937.
15. Witzel MA, Clarke JA, Lindsay WK, Thomson HG. Comparison of results of pushback or von Langenbeck repair of isolated cleft of the hard and soft palate. Plast Reconstr Surg. 1979; 64: 347–52.
16. Bardach J, Salyer KE. Cleft palate repair. In Bardach J, Salyer KE (Eds.): Surgical Techniques in Cleft Lip and Palate. St. Louis, MO: Mosby, 1991.
17. Gillett DA, Clarke HM. The hybrid palatoplasty: a preliminary report. Can J Plast Surg. 1996; 4: 157–60.
18. Mahoney MH, Fisher DM. An audit of primary palatoplasty: One surgeon/485 cases/10 years. Paper presented at: 64th Annual Meeting of the Canadian Society of Plastic Surgeons; June 15–19, 2010; Halifax, Nova Scotia, Canada.
19. Sommerlad BC. A technique for cleft palate repair. Plast Reconstr Surg. 2003; 112: 1542–8.
20. Sommerlad BC. Cleft palate. In Guyuron B, Eriksson E, Persing J (Eds.): Plastic Surgery. Philadelphia: Saunders, 2009.
21. Sommerlad BC. Cleft palate repair. In Losee JE, Kirschner R (Eds.): Comprehensive Cleft Care. New York: McGraw-Hill, 2009.
22. Furlow LT Jr. Cleft palate repair by double opposing Z-plasty. Plast Reconstr Surg. 1986; 78: 724–38.
23. Furlow LT. Cleft palate repair by double opposing Z-plasty. Oper Tech Plast Reconstr Surg. 1995; 2: 223–30.
24. LaRossa D, Hunenko-Jackson O, Kirschner RE, et al. The Children's Hospital of Philadelphia modification of the Furlow double opposing Z-plasty: long-term speech and growth results. Clin Plast Surg. 2004; 31: 243–9.
25. Armour A, Fischbach S, Klaiman P, Fisher DM. Does velopharyngeal closure pattern affect the success of pharyngeal flap pharyngoplasty? Plast Reconstr Surg. 2005; 115: 45–52; discussion 53.
26. Sommerlad BC, Henley M, Birch M, et al. Cleft palate re-repair: a clinical and radiological study of 32 consecutive cases. Br J Plast Surg. 1994; 47: 406–10.
27. Sommerlad BC, Mehendale FV, Birch MJ, et al. Palate re-repair re-visited. Cleft Palate J. 2002; 39: 295–307.

28. Hynes W. Pharyngoplasty by muscle transplantation. Br J Plast Surg. 1950; 3: 128–35.

29. Moss AL, Pigott RW, Albery EH. Hynes pharyngoplasty revisited. Plast Reconstr Surg. 1987; 79: 346–55.

30. Sommerlad BC. The use of an operating microscope in cleft palate repair and pharyngoplasty. Plast Reconstr Surg. 2003; 112: 1540–1.

31. Becker M, Hansson E. Low rate of fistula formation after Sommerlad palatoplasty with or without lateral incisions: an analysis of risk factors for formation of fistulas after palatoplasty. J Plast Reconstr Aesthet Surg. 2013; 66: 697–703.

32. Moar KK, Sweet C, Beale V. Fistula rate after primary palatal repair with intravelarveloplasty: a retrospective three-year audit of six units (NorCleft) in the UK. Br J Oral Maxillofac Surg. 2016; 54: 634–7.

33. Téblick S, Ruymaekers M, Van de Casteele E, Nadjmi N. Effect of cleft palate closure technique on speech and middle ear outcome: a systematic review. J Oral Maxillofac Surg. 2019; 77: 405.e1–e15.

CHAPTER 17

Alveolar Cleft Bone Grafting (Part II): Secondary Bone Grafting

Ochs MW. J Oral Maxillofac Surg. 1996; 54: 83–8.

Reviewed by John Rowson, David Grimes and Cristina Frezzini

Research Question/Objective

Review of alveolar bone grafting (ABG) techniques for alveolar clefts. Areas reviewed were timing, graft materials and donor site. Key published papers up to the time of publication were reviewed.

Study Design

This is a clinical review article from a single surgeon.

This review highlighted that ABG should provide a continuous and stable maxillary alveolus, without oronasal fistulae, with alar base support, bone for tooth eruption and orthodontic movement into the site, or potential dental implant placement.

It is suggested that dental development rather than age should be the primary determinant of timing, usually focusing on the developmental stage of the permanent maxillary canine.

Autogenous bone grafting is seen as the material of choice, with there being advantages and disadvantages for each potential donor site, which should therefore be discussed and decided upon with the patient.

Relevant Studies

This paper is a review of the current practice at the time of publication.[1]

Not a great deal has changed in the meantime, but there are some areas where alternative methods may now be considered.

Timing

There has been controversy about the timing of ABG for some years.[1-3] The current consensus seems to have moved to secondary ABG that is carried out after 2 years old and timed to assist eruption of the secondary maxillary dentition.

Commonly this is to accommodate the maxillary canine but surgery may done be earlier to accommodate the lateral incisor in some patients and there are a small number of centres who prefer earlier grafting at about 6 years as a routine. In the United Kingdom the consensus is to coincide with eruption of the canine or, where indicated, the lateral incisor.[4] Most sources agree that delay until adulthood is to be avoided if possible although there will be exceptions where this becomes necessary.

The decision to graft is taken by the Multi-Disciplinary Team (cleft MDT) with the orthodontist often the key opinion. Most centres aim to graft when the canine root is half to two thirds formed.

There may be social, personal, or other clinical reasons that affect the timing, however, so an MDT assessment is always recommended.

The stated aims of ABG are well known and include bony continuity, support for the eruption of teeth, closure of oronasal communication, support for the nasal ala, improved arch form, gingival contour and to support maxillary growth. Some sources include preparation for implants but this is often difficult and an onlay graft for implants is sometimes required at a later date.[1]

Surgically this requires meticulous dissection and closure of the nasal and oral mucosa and placement of a cancellous bone graft.[1]

Imaging to Assess Results

In the United Kingdom, units providing cleft surgery are expected to record a Kindelan score for all patients with a unilateral cleft lip and palate 6 months after an alveolar bone graft.[5] This requires an anterior occlusal radiograph to be taken 6 months postoperatively. Whether this guides further treatment or provides prognostic information is not well evidenced.

The availability of cone beam CT (CBCT) has led to attempts to provide protocols for this modality of imaging for ABG planning and measurement of success. These protocols have little evidence for or against the use of CBCT although it is likely to prove useful for research.

Postoperative assessment by CBCT may give a better volumetric assessment; however, the benefit of three-dimensional imaging needs to be weighed against the risk of an increase in radiation exposure. Although total dose radiation exposure with CBCT is relatively low, it is still higher than when using plain upper occlusal radiographs.

De Mulder et al.[6] compared radiation exposure for ABG assessment using panoramic radiograph as a baseline for exposure. The CBCT manufacturer was not described but they defined the requirements for imaging as low resolution with a field of view of 8 cm by 5 cm to reduce exposure of radiosensitive tissue such as the lens of the eye or the thyroid gland. With these precautions they calculated the CBCT exposed the patient to four to six times the dose compared to a panoramic radiograph (an absolute exposure of 3–4.5 days of background radiation).

This would suggest that until the radiation dose is more in line with that of plain radiographs, the latter will be first choice for imaging unless specific indications (such as establishing the presence of root resorption or position or number of supernumerary teeth) exist.[7,8]

Material-Future Perspectives

Both autologous and alloplastic materials have been used as the source of bone for ABG in alveolar cleft.[9] Autologous bone still represents the gold standard for bone regeneration, because of its known osteogenic and osteoconductive potential. Bone is most commonly harvested from a patient's iliac crest, mandible, or tibia, and the choice of donor site is influenced by many factors including surgeon experience and volume of the alveolar defect. Other donor sites are described but rarely used. Often the graft is entirely cancellous bone, although some advocate cortico-cancellous blocks but there is no evidence that this gives significantly better results.[1,10]

The use of a suitable allogenic material would negate morbidity of the donor site in ABG although in experienced hands donor site morbidity is low.[11]

Recombinant human morphogenic protein 2 (rh-BMP2) has been investigated as suitable alternative to autologous bone. A recent systematic review with meta-analysis identified five randomised controlled trials (RCTs) comparing iliac bone graft with rh-BMP2 in ABG, evaluated at 6 months and 1 year with CT evaluation. In these studies, rh-BMP2 provided higher volume of bone compared to iliac bone at 6 months, although this difference was not maintained at 1 year. Iliac crest and rh-BMP2 provided similar bone graft height at 6 months.[12]

The addition of bone shaving from the zygoma to the use of rh-BMP2 appears to provide a further advantage in the efficiency of bone formation when compared to iliac bone graft or rh-BMP2 alone.[12]

The advantages of using allogenic material have been reported to be lack of donor site morbidity, decreased postoperative pain (which is reported to be more significant in the donor site than in the alveolar area) and possibly decreased hospital stay. Thus far, therefore, the absence of a significant difference between autologous bone graft and rh-BMP2 graft in terms of bone volume and height at the ABG site offers a promising alternative method of alveolar reconstruction in ABG patients.

REFERENCES

1. Ochs MW. Alveolar cleft bone grafting (Part II): secondary bone grafting. J Oral Maxillofac Surg. 1996; 54: 83–8.
2. Dissaux C, Bodin F, Grollemund B, et al. Evaluation of success of alveolar cleft bone graft performed at 5 years versus 10 years of age. J Oral Maxillofac Surg. 2016; 44: 21–6.
3. Siegenthaler M, Bettelini L, Brudnicki A, Rachwalski M, Fudalej PS. Early versus late alveolar bone grafting in unilateral cleft lip and palate: dental arch relationships in pre-adolescent patients. J Oral Maxillofac Surg. 2018; 46: 2052–7.
4. Colbert SD, Green B, Brennan PA, Mercer N. Contemporary management of cleft lip and palate in the United Kingdom. Have we reached the turning point? Br J Oral Maxillofac Surg. 2015; 53: 594–8.
5. Kindelan JD, Nashed RR, Bromige MR. Radiographic assessment of secondary autogenous alveolar bone grafting in cleft lip and palate patients. Cleft Palate Craniofac J. 1997; 34: 195–8.
6. De Mulder D, Cadenas de Llano-Pérula M, Willems G, et al. An optimized imaging protocol for orofacial cleft patients. Clin Exp Dent Res. 2018; 4: 152–7.
7. Oenning AC, Jacobs R, Pauwels R, et al. DIMITRA research group. Cone-beam CT in paediatric dentistry: DIMITRA project position statement. Pediatr Radiol. 2018; 48: 308–16.
8. Horner K, Islam M, Flygare L, Tsiklakis K, Whaites E. Basic principles for use of dental cone beam computed tomography: consensus guidelines of the European academy of dental and maxillofacial radiology. Dentomaxillofac Radiol. 2009; 38: 187–95.
9. Scalzone A, Flores-Mir C, Carozza D, et al. Secondary alveolar bone grafting using autologous versus alloplastic material in the treatment of cleft lip and palate patients: systematic review and meta-analysis. Prog Orthod. 2019; 20: 6.
10. Demas PN, Sotereanos GC. Closure of alveolar clefts with corticocancellous block grafts and marrow: a retrospective study. J Oral Maxillofac Surg. 1988; 46: 682–7.
11. Brudnicki A, Rachwalski M, Wiepszowski Ł, Sawicka E. Secondary alveolar bone grafting in cleft lip and palate: a comparative analysis of donor site morbidity in different age groups. J Craniomaxillofac Surg. 2019; 47: 165–9.
12. Balaj SM. Alveolar cleft defect closure with iliac bone graft, rhBMP-2 and rhBMP-2 with zygoma shavings: comparative study. Ann Maxillofac Surg. 2011; 1: 8–13.

CHAPTER **18**

Timing of Treatment for Craniosynostosis and Faciocraniosynostosis: A 20-Year Experience

Marchac D, Renier D, Broumand S. Br J Plast Surg. 1994; 47: 211–22.

Reviewed by Jennifer Vesey and Ben Robertson

Research Question/Objective

The objective of the paper was to discuss the treatment protocols for, and timing of, surgery in patients with craniosynostosis treated at the Hôpital Necker-Enfants Malades, Paris, France. The paper reflects on the author's experience in performing surgery for single suture and complex craniofacial conditions over a 20-year period.

Study Design

This was a review paper of the management of patients with craniofacial synostosis. The authors specifically mention that this is not an outcome-based paper but a reflection on their experience and details their treatment protocols for the various craniofacial suture synostoses.

Sample Size

This paper reflects on a cohort population of 1,247 patients with craniosynostosis, of which 987 received surgical intervention. Since the time of publication (1994) to present day, it has been one of the largest studies of craniofacial patients reported on in the literature.

Follow-up

Not applicable.

Inclusion/Exclusion Criteria

The paper discussed the author's experience in the management of patients with syndromic and non-syndromic craniosynostosis who were operated in between 1973 and 1993, by one team at the Hôpital Necker-Enfants Malades, Paris.

Intervention or Treatment Received

Patients received surgical treatment for their craniosynostosis according to their age at referral and the protocols of the unit. The paper outlines different

treatment approaches for the full range of craniosynostoses and discusses each
of them in turn.

Results

The authors' ideal timings and treatment approaches for the various
craniosynostoses were outlined and summarised. They described the different
protocols they used when patients were referred for treatment early, slightly
delayed, moderately delayed and late, and the principles behind these.

In patients who presented early with non-syndromic craniosynostosis or
brachycephaly, treatment was undertaken according to the protocol outlined
in Table 18.1. The authors reported that up to 2 years of age, there was
little difference in the management of craniosynostosis except for patients
with brachycephaly (Table 18.1). The change in protocol for patients with
brachycephaly was due to the reduced potential for postoperative brain
expansion after 6 months of age. They advised that between 2 and 5 years old
the same surgical techniques can be utilised; however, the bone is more difficult
to cut and mould, and breaks easily. Additionally, it is not possible to rely on
spontaneous re-ossification and complete reconstruction is recommended.

Once the patient reaches 5 years old, there are two additional considerations
that need to be taken into account: facial malformations and development of
the frontal sinus. The facial malformations highlighted were those of patients
with plagiocephaly where asymmetry of the affected orbit and deviation of the
nose often require surgical intervention and trigonocephaly where narrowing
of the face may be obvious and managed by moving the orbital walls, and

Table 18.1 The timing of treatment for craniosynostosis (adapted from Marchac et al.[1])

Condition	2–4 Months	4–6 Months	6–9 Months	1–2 Years	2–6 Years	6–12 Years	12–18 Years
Brachycephaly	Floating forehead	Forehead advancement using tongue in groove					
Trigonocephaly			Frontocranial remodelling				
Plagiocephaly			Frontocranial remodelling		Frontocranial remodelling (more difficult procedure)	Frontocranial remodelling + frontal sinuses	Forehead, orbit + nasal correction
Scaphocephaly	Parasagittal craniectomies		Frontocranial remodelling				
Pancraniosynostosis	Release + reconstruction with pieces		Frontocranial remodelling				
Turricephaly			Anterior + posterior remodelling				
Oxycephaly				Frontocranial remodelling			
Apert syndrome	Floating forehead advancement		Forehead advancement using tongue in groove			Le Fort III	Le Fort I
Crouzon syndrome							

occasionally the zygomatic areas, laterally. When the frontal sinus is present the authors advised that the upper part, which is included in the supra-orbital bar, is removed, the mucosa elevated, and the posterior wall resected. They found that the frontal sinus will develop again in most patients operated on before 8 years old.

In patients with Apert's or Crouzon's syndrome a floating forehead advancement was the approach of choice between 2 and 4 months old and a forehead advancement with tongue in groove after 6 months. If there was severe exorbitism, then a Monobloc advancement was recommended. However, it was noted this was associated with a higher infection risk. Correction of the midface was undertaken after 6 years old in a two-stage process. Ideally, the facial advancement is delayed until the permanent dentition and a stable occlusion can be achieved.

The authors described more unusual situations in which alternative approaches may be required. These included multi-suture craniosynostoses, patients with brain malformations, and those with craniosynostoses and hydrocephalus. They felt that in patients with multi-sutural synostoses at risk of severe brain constriction and raised intracranial pressure, the surgery should be undertaken as soon as possible, depending on the condition of the patient. Surgical management should aim to reposition the supra-orbital bar in a normal position so that the upper forehead is well contoured. The remaining bony pieces are positioned loosely on the rest of the vault with the brain to act as a natural expander. In patients with anomalies due to brain malformation, functional prognosis is not as good. Where the brain is not obviously constricted, surgery is delayed until 3–9 months of age. The authors highlighted the complexities in the timing of treatment for patients with craniosynostosis and hydrocephalus due to the potential for "dead space" to be created, and subsequent complications related to this, if treated concurrently. They advised assessment on a case by case basis.

Study Limitations

This is a review paper that includes authors expert opinions based on their experiences and therefore falls at the lower end of the hierarchy of evidence. However, due to the relatively low incidence of craniosynostosis, there are limited high-volume studies and this was among the best evidence available at the time the paper was published. The paper was published in 1994 (26 years ago) and since then, there have been many advancements in techniques for the surgical management of craniosynostosis. The techniques discussed are not necessarily contemporaneous with current clinical practice. Advances in genetics also mean that many of the non-syndromic craniosynostoses cases included in this review would likely be reclassified as syndromic craniosynostoses.

Relevant Studies

This was a seminal paper describing the techniques used in the management of patients with syndromic and non-syndromic craniosynostosis. While many of the principles outlined still hold true, a number of changes have occurred in philosophy and treatment modalities since it was published, mostly due to newer operative techniques and equipment.

The biggest changes have arisen due to the introduction of distraction osteogenesis as a treatment modality. Posterior vault distraction has become the mainstay for early surgical expansion of skull volume. This technique, pioneered by the Birmingham Craniofacial Unit, utilises distraction osteogenesis to push the posterior skull backwards, allowing for a significant increase in volume compared to fronto-orbital advancement and remodelling (FOAR).[2] This technique decreases the raised intracranial pressure associated with multi-suture synostosis as well as improving/minimising chiari malformations and syrinxes.[3]

Posterior vault distraction is now the treatment choice for bicoronal synostosis in patients with a known syndrome (Apert, Crouzon, etc.) or those bicoronal conditions yet to be genetically diagnosed. This then aims to also prevent the turri-brachycephaly/oxycephaly that is so difficult to treat by FOAR. The added benefit of this technique is due to Newton's third law, with some improvement in forehead position often achieved. Often though, a FOAR is still required to normalise the pre-existing skeletal abnormality. In patients with Apert or Crouzon (and sometimes Pfeiffer) syndrome, significant midface retrusion occurs. This has implications for breathing, sleep, dental occlusion, and appearance. Marchac's (and Tessier's) philosophy on performing a FOAR with midface advancement at a delayed stage compared to Ortiz-Monasterio's monobloc technique is still valid today. There are benefits and negatives to both techniques and should be applied to each individual patient.

The other major change from Marchac's philosophy again relates to distraction osteogenesis. Advancement of the midface (using either a Le Fort 3 osteotomy or a Monobloc osteotomy), is increasingly performed with distraction osteogenesis as this technique has been shown to significantly reduce the risk of infection and relapse associated with previous techniques.[4]

REFERENCES

1. Marchac D, Renier D, Broumand S. Timing of treatment for craniosynostosis and faciocraniosynostosis: a 20-year experience. Br J Plast Surg. 1994; 47: 211–22.
2. White N, Evans M, Dover MS, et al. Posterior calvarial vault expansion using distraction osteogenesis. Childs Nerv Syst. 2009; 25: 231–6.
3. Lin LO, Zhang RS, Hoppe IC, et al. Onset and resolution of Chiari malformations and hydrocephalus in syndromic craniosynostosis following posterior vault distraction. Plast Reconstr Surg. 2019; 144: 932–40.

CHAPTER 19

Lengthening the Human Mandible by Gradual Distraction

McCarthy JG, Schreiber J, Karp N, Thorne CH, Grayson BH.
Plast Reconstr Surg. 1992; 89: 1–8.

Reviewed by David M McGoldrick and Kevin McMillan

Research Question/Objective

Distraction osteogenesis in long limbs was shown by a Ilizarov and others in the 1980s to be an efficacious and safe procedure.[1] Although the application of this technique demonstrated stable lengthening in the canine mandible, no previous human studies had been published prior to this paper.[2,3] This study was essentially a proof of concept study in humans.

Study Design/Sample Size

The paper reports a case series of four patients. All patients were male with an age range between 23 and 131 months. Three cases involved unilateral distraction and in the fourth, the technique was applied bilaterally.

Follow-up

Patients were followed up at 6-month intervals. Photographs, radiographs and dental models were recorded at the end of the distraction period and at these 6 month intervals. Follow-up for the patients ranged from 11 to 20 months.

Intervention

The mandibular distraction was applied by a novel external calibrated device. The surgical technique involved exposure of the mandible via a Risdon (submandibular) approach followed by supra-periosteal dissection. Two bi-cortical pins were placed at 10 mm and 14 mm distances on each side of a proposed corticotomy. The corticotomy was then performed using a drill and osteotomes.

A 7-day latent period was employed after surgery, before activation of the device. After this, the segments were expanded by 1 mm per day for 20 days. At the completion of the distraction phase, the expansion was maintained for 9 weeks before device removal.

Results

The authors reported a mean expansion of 20 mm with a range of 18–24 mm. Patients were maintained in external fixation for an average of 9 weeks and no perioperative complications were reported.

The first patient was treated at 23 months for right hemifacial microsomia. An expansion of 18 mm was achieved which was stable at 17 months. The second patient underwent bilateral distraction at age 8 years and 2 months for Nager syndrome. Expansions of 24 mm and 22 mm respectively were achieved; however, a relapse of 5 mm was reported at 9 months. The patient, the oldest treated, reported normal lip sensation, although their scars were deemed to be unsatisfactory.

The third case involved a child with left hemifacial microsomia treated at 5 years 1 month of age. Expansion of 20 mm was achieved which was stable at 9 months. The patient fell on the device during treatment, but there were no complications reported. The final patient was treated at 10 years and 11 months for left hemifacial microsomia. They also achieved 20 mm of expansion that was stable at follow-up.

Limitations

The major limitation of this paper is that it is a heterogeneous case series of four patients with varying ages and pathology. Although the reported follow-up demonstrated good stability, the overall timeframe for follow-up is short when potential confounding factors such as growth are considered.

Relevant Studies

This landmark paper has been widely cited since its original publication over 25 years ago. The strength of the paper is demonstrated by the widespread adoption of the technique by craniofacial surgeons, and it has formed the basis for developments in mandibular distraction.

The 1990s saw a number of other units publish on their experience of this technique with similar results.[4–6] This period also saw the technique evolve with the development of firstly bi-directional and then multi-directional devices.[7,8] These devices aimed to improve both functional and structural results in patients with both skeletal deficiency and malocclusion. The subsequent development of intra-oral devices was also a major evolution with greatly improved patient acceptability.[9]

Mandibular distraction has also evolved as a reliable technique for use in cases of pediatric airway obstruction. The technique has been employed successfully in paediatric patients with craniofacial abnormalities such as Pierre Robin sequence, reducing tracheostomy requirements in up to 80–90% of cases.[10–12] Although the technique has been used in children with Treacher Collins syndrome, it is now recognised that it should be combined with midface distraction and rotation to maximise airway decompression.[13]

One criticism of this paper was the relatively short follow-up time, giving rise to concerns about the long-term stability of the procedure. The main initial proponents of the technique later published their long-term results demonstrating effectiveness and stability in their cohorts.[14–16] The authors acknowledged, however, that not all outcomes are satisfactory and that age at intervention and degrees of overcorrection are important variables.

Conversely, some authors have questioned the long-term benefits of the technique and the common requirement for orthognathic treatment in later life.[17,18] Indeed one recent comparative study showed no difference in rates of orthognathic surgery between those who underwent distraction and those who did not.[19] These authors do however accept that benefits are likely to exist in terms of bone stock for later surgery, soft tissue growth profile and the psychological effect on patients. Overall evidence for this technique remains of a relatively low level and on-going work will be required to further determine the optimal timing and indications for this procedure.

Since the initial demonstration for use of distraction osteogenesis of the mandible in congenital craniofacial deformities, its use in other areas of the facial skeleton and for other congenital and acquired facial deformities has expanded markedly.[20–24] As with mandibular distraction, there remains questions about optimal indications, technique and timing.

REFERENCES

1. Ilizarov GA, Devyatov AA, Kamerin VK. Plastic reconstruction of longitudinal bone defects by means of compression and subsequent distraction. Acta Chir Plast. 1980; 22: 32–41.
2. Snyder CC, Levine GA, Swanson HM, Browne EZ. Mandibular lengthening by gradual distraction: preliminary report. Plast Reconstr Surg. 1973; 51: 506–8.
3. Karp NS, Thorne CHM, McCarthy JG, Sissons HA. Bone lengthening on the craniofacial skeleton. Ann Plast Surg. 1990; 24: 231–7.
4. Kollar EM, Diner PA, Vazquez MP, Accart G, Pirollo M. Bone distraction using an external fixator: a new mandibular lengthening technic. A preliminary study apropos of 2 cases of children with mandibular hypoplasia. [Article in French]. Rev Stomatol Chir Maxillofac. 1994; 95: 411–6.
5. Rachmiel A, Levy M, Laufer D. Lengthening of the mandible by distraction osteogenesis: report of cases. J Oral Maxillofac Surg. 1995; 53: 838–46.
6. Havlik RJ, Bartlett SP. Mandibular distraction lengthening in the severely hypoplastic mandible: a problematic case with tongue aplasia. J Craniofac Surg. 1994; 5: 305–10.

7. Molina F, Ortiz Monasterio F. Mandibular elongation and remodeling by distraction: a farewell to major osteotomies. Plast Reconstr Surg. 1995; 96: 825–40.

8. McCarthy JG, Williams JK, Grayson BH, Crombie JS. Controlled multiplanar distraction of the mandible: device development and clinical application. J Craniofac Surg. 1998; 9: 322–9.

9. Diner PA, Kollar EM, Martinez H, Vazquez MP. Intraoral distraction for mandibular lengthening: a technical innovation. J Craniomaxillofac Surg. 1996; 24: 92–5.

10. Moore MH, Guzman-Stein G, Proudman TW, et al. Mandibular lengthening by distraction for airway obstruction in Treacher-Collins syndrome. J Craniofac Surg. 1994 Feb; 5: 22–5.

11. Genecov DG, Barcelo CR, Steinberg D, Trone T, Sperry E. Clinical experience with the application of distraction osteogenesis for airway obstruction. J Craniofac Surg. 2009; 20: 1817–21.

12. Tahiri Y, Viezel-Mathieu A, Aldekhayel S, Lee J, Gilardino M. The effectiveness of mandibular distraction in improving airway obstruction in the pediatric population. Plast Reconstr Surg. 2014; 133: 352e–9e.

13. Hopper RA, Kapadia H, Susarla S, Bly R, Johnson K. Counterclockwise craniofacial distraction osteogenesis for tracheostomy-dependent children with Treacher Collins Syndrome. Plast Reconstr Surg. 2018; 142: 447–57.

14. Molina F. Mandibular distraction osteogenesis: a clinical experience of the last 17 years. J Craniofac Surg. 2009; 20: 1794–800.

15. Shetye PR, Grayson BH, Mackool RJ, McCarthy JG. Long-term stability and growth following unilateral mandibular distraction in growing children with craniofacial microsomia. Plast Reconstr Surg. 2006; 118: 985–95.

16. Weichman KE, Jacobs J, Patel P, et al. Early distraction for mild to moderate unilateral craniofacial microsomia: long-term follow-Up, outcomes, and recommendations. Plast Reconstr Surg. 2017; 139: 941e–53e.

17. Nagy K, Kuijpers-Jagtman AM, Mommaerts MY. No evidence for long-term effectiveness of early osteodistraction in hemifacial microsomia. Plast Reconstr Surg. 2009; 124: 2061–71.

18. Ascenço AS, Balbinot P, Junior IM, et al. Mandibular distraction in hemifacial microsomia is not a permanent treatment: a long-term evaluation. J Craniofac Surg. 2014; 25: 352–4.

19. Zhang RS, Lin LO, Hoppe IC, et al. Early mandibular distraction in craniofacial microsomia and need for orthognathic correction at skeletal maturity: a comparative long-term follow-up study. Plast Reconstr Surg. 2018; 142: 1285–93.

20. Hidding J, Lazar F, Zoller JE. Initial outcome of vertical distraction osteogenesis of the atrophic alveolar ridge. Mund Kiefer Gesichtschir. 1993; 3: 79–83.

21. Stucki-McCormick SU, Fox R, Mizrahi R, Ericksom M. Transport distraction: mandibular reconstruction. Atlas Oral Maxillofac Clin N Am. 1999; 7: 65–84.

22. Stucki-McCormick SU, Fox RM, Mizrahi RD. Reconstruction of a neocondyle using transport distraction osteogenesis. Semin Orthod. 1999; 5: 59–63.

23. White N, Evans M, Dover MS, Noons P, Solanki G, Nishikawa H. Posterior calvarial vault expansion using distraction osteogenesis. Childs Nerv Syst 2009; 25: 231–236.

24. Cohen SR. Midface distraction. Semin Orthod. 1999; 116: 264–70.

25. Klesper B, Lazar F, Siessegger M, et al. Vertical distraction osteogenesis of fibula transplants for mandibular reconstruction—a preliminary study. J Craniomaxillofac Surg. 2002; 30: 280–5.

CHAPTER 20

Advancement of the Orbits and the Midface in One Piece, Combined with Frontal Repositioning, for the Correction of Crouzon's Deformities

Ortiz-Monasterio F, Fuente del Campo A, Carillo A.
Plast Reconstr Surg. 1978; 61: 507–16.

Reviewed by Günter Lauer

Research Question/Objective

This is the first report on the surgical technique of cranio-orbito-facial monobloc advancement in Crouzon's disease to correct a severe facial malformation.

Study Design

Single-centre case-based study introducing the surgical technique of combined fronto-orbito-facial advancement (FOFA) as a single-step procedure. In general, the craniofacial unit of the authors has extensive experience in orbital and facial mobilisation, stemming from 176 cases, 71 of them suffering from Crouzon's and Apert's syndromes. Here, a newly developed operative technique is presented and the first results of the clinical follow-up are reported in the form of a retrospective study.

Sample Size

In total, seven patients suffering from Crouzon's deformity were operated on; five children aged between 4 and 6 years and two adults aged 24 and 35 years.

Follow-up

Follow-up was variable, up to 3 years, and the authors comment that further follow-up is required to assess growth in the children.

Inclusion/Exclusion Criteria

Only patients suffering from Crouzon's syndrome were included; other syndromes particularly Apert's syndrome cases were excluded.

Intervention or Treatment Received

In these seven patients, an orbito-facial monobloc advancement combined with a frontal/cranial advancement was performed to correct the cranial and facial malformation simultaneously. To stabilise the monobloc in its anterior position, different sources of bone grafts (hip, rib, skull) were interposed into the gaps created and fixed with wire sutures.

Results

A satisfactory postoperative course is reported in all patients, with no serious complications such as cerebro-spinal fluid (CSF) fistula, frontal bone flap loss, or meningitis. Postoperatively the dental occlusion remained normal in four patients, two followed-up for 3 years, one for 2 years and one for 1 year. Exorbitism was corrected in all cases, giving a more anatomical correction than previous techniques due to simultaneous advancement of the whole orbital ring.

Study Limitations

The study shows that the FOFA–monobloc technique is feasible to advance the frontal cranium, the orbits, and the midface simultaneously, but the number of patients reported here is small, and the results of later studies with bigger numbers of patients and longer follow-up periods are not as good.[1]

Relevant Studies

The correction of craniofacial midface malformations has undergone considerable development over the last decades to improve/correct problems associated with function such as breathing, vision, food intake, and chewing, as well as with aesthetics and the patient's psychosocial well-being. More than 60 years ago, Gillies and Harrison described the surgical correction of the orbits and the midface in the case of a young woman.[2] In 1969, Obwegeser described different osteotomy levels to approach and surgically correct small and retrodisplaced maxillae, and in 1971 Tessier published a series of cases describing the intracranial approach to correct midface dysplasia and hypertelorism.[3,4]

In syndromic facial dysplasia, however, the cranium is involved as well as the midface. Ortiz-Monasterio and colleagues have here described the FOFA as a monobloc procedure in a series of seven patients, thus correcting frontal and midface deformities in a single step in patients suffering from Crouzon.

Later studies with larger numbers and longer follow-up demonstrated higher complication rates, including CSF leakage, frontal bone flap loss, and infection due to the space created between the brain and the monobloc and the communication between the nasal sinuses and the brain/meninges.[1]

In order to overcome the problem of ascending infection, a galeo-pericranial flap combined with bone grafts to cover the skull base defect has been described.[5]

Given the limited stability of the fixation technique available at the time, with wires and bone grafts, the complication rate, with only one patient losing part of the frontal bone, was excellent. Although there are no studies specifically considering whether miniplate osteosynthesis has reduced complication rates, this has become normal practice.

There are several papers that discuss the advantages and disadvantages of a two-stage approach (FOA first, LeFort III later) versus the FOFA monobloc.[6,7] Factors that influence whether to use the monobloc or two-stage approach are age and impairment of function due the malformation of the midface.[8] Even in craniofacial centres, there is a high complication rate of CSF leak, loss of the frontal bone flap, or sequestration of bone grafts in more than 30% of cases with FOFA monobloc procedures.[9] Consequently, the recommendation to perform a monobloc procedure was limited to where there was a risk to the eyes, and for breathing impairment at an age more than 3 years.[10]

Another significant change in the operative approach to craniofacial malformation has been the advent of distraction osteogenesis (DO). Polley et al. first reported using DO on a newborn to correct the midface, thus allowing globe and corneal protection and airway patency.[11] Since then surgical techniques for DO have been further refined, and where extraoral distractors devices were necessary in the beginning,[12] it is now possible to use several subcutaneous distractors at the same time to direct more precisely the advancement of the complete monobloc.[13]

With quadruple distraction techniques, adjustment of the distraction vector is possible, leading to improved results in the position of the midface.[13,14] In particular, Arnaud et al.[9] showed prospectively that with four internal distractors (quadruple internal distraction), FOFA can reliably correct respiratory impairment and exophthalmos even in young patients suffering from syndromic facio-craniosynostosis, with significantly reduced complications such as CSF leakage and frontal bone infection.

Bradley et al.[14] compared complication rates and relapse of advancement applying three different types of monobloc advancement: conventional advancement, conventional advancement combined with a pericranial flap to seal off the skull base, and monobloc advancement by distraction osteogenesis. The complication rate was lowest after distraction (8%) and highest after conventional advancement without pericranial flap (61%). Further, the relapse was lowest after distraction using only two distractors and adjustment of the occlusion achieved via elastics and occlusion screws.[9,14] With all of these adjustments, distraction osteogenesis can allow a monobloc approach with complication rates comparable to a two-step approach.

The timing for monobloc advancement by distraction has been discussed extensively. Early papers recommending FOFA at an early point in life, around 7 months,[15] while later papers and summaries advocate for FOFA surgery as late as possible—3 years onwards, and only in severest risks of globe cornea damage and breathing impairment is surgery recommended at an earlier point. In cases of raised intracranial pressure at a very early age, recent papers recommend early pressure relief by a posterior cranioplasty and postponing a FOFA as late as possible.[16,17]

If in addition to anterior advancement, transverse changes in the naso-orbito-ethmoidal region are necessary, bone resection in the central fronto-nasal area is possible. In a facial bipartition a central piece of bone in fronto-nasal area is resected and the lateral bone margins brought together so that the frontal bone as well as the zygomatic area becomes narrower.[18] The orbital frames may also be repositioned separately, depending on the type of malformation.[19] These techniques allow for hypertelorism to be corrected without detachment and reinsertion of the medial canthal ligament. If there is deformity of the naso-orbito-ethmoidal area (Figure 20.1) such as with fronto-ethmoidal meningo-encephaloceles, Pinzer et al. described a series of nearly sixty patients where reliable correction of the hypertelorism/ telecanthus was achieved by bone resection in the orbito-naso-ethmoid and infraorbital region combined with detachment and consecutive reinsertion of the medial canthal ligament. (Figure 20.2).[20] Interestingly, using their fixation technique for the medial canthal ligament, telecanthus as well as hypertelorism improved in the still growing face. To make the outcome more predictable and reliable,

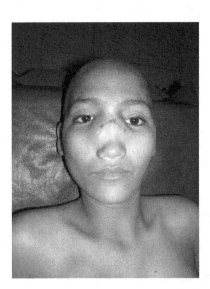

Figure 20.1   Fourteen-year-old girl with telecanthus suffering from fronto-orbital meningoencephalocele prior to surgery.

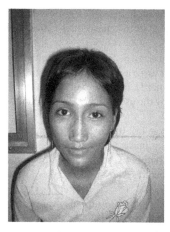

Figure 20.2 The girl 6 months after surgery. The telecanthus has been improved considerably after resection of the meningoencephalocele using a transcrauncular suture.

intraoperative navigation and imaging as well as preoperative planning using three-dimensional (3-D) models have already had an additional impact. With intraoperative navigation the position of the cutting device can be controlled during surgery.[21] Virtual planning and 3-D models of the patients may be used to check the placement of the distractor device, osteotomy design, and the vector to move the monobloc segment.[22] Finally, the intraoperative navigation can be used to double-check whether the preoperatively planned result was achieved intraoperatively.[23]

In general, this paper widened the surgical horizons to approach the transitional area between midface and cranial bone. Besides malformation surgery, it also has a significant impact on the approach to the skull base area in trauma- and ablative oncologic surgery.

REFERENCES

1. Fearon JA, Whitaker LA. Complications with facial advancement: a comparison between the Le Fort III and monobloc advancements. Plast Reconstr Surg. 1993; 91: 990–5.
2. Gillies H, Harrison SH. Operative correction by osteotomy of recessed malar maxillary compound in a case of oxycephaly. Br J Plast Surg. 1950; 3: 123–7.
3. Obwegeser HL. Surgical correction of small or retrodisplaced maxillae. The "dish-face" deformity. Plast Reconstr Surg. 1969; 43: 351–65.
4. Tessier P. The definitive plastic surgical treatment of the severe facial deformities of craniofacial dysostosis. Crouzon's and Apert's diseases. Plast Reconstr Surg. 1971; 48: 419–42.
5. Lee Y, Kim WJ. How to make the blockage between the nasal cavity and intracranial space using a four-layer sealing technique. Plast Reconstr Surg. 2006; 117: 233–8.
6. McCarthy JG, Epstein F, Sadove M, Grayson B, Zide B. Early surgery for craniofacial synostosis: an 8-year experience. Plast Reconstr Surg. 1984; 73: 521–33.

7. Whitaker LA, Bartlett SP, Schut L, Bruce D. Craniosynostosis: an analysis of the timing, treatment, and complications in 164 consecutive patients. Plast Reconstr Surg. 1987; 80: 195–212.

8. Marchac D, Renier D, Broumand S. Timing of treatment for craniosynostosis and facio-craniosynostosis: a 20-year experience. Br J Plast Surg. 1994; 47: 211–22.

9. Arnaud E, Marchac D, Renier D. Reduction of morbidity of the frontofacial monobloc advancement in children by the use of internal distraction. Plast Reconstr Surg. 2007; 120: 1009–26.

10. Wolfe SA1, Morrison G, Page LK, Berkowitz S. The monobloc frontofacial advancement: do the pluses outweigh the minuses? Plast Reconstr Surg. 1993; 91: 977–87.

11. Polley JW, Figueroa AA, Charbel FT, et al. Monobloc craniomaxillofacial distraction osteogenesis in a newborn with severe craniofacial synostosis: a preliminary report. J Craniofac Surg. 1995; 6: 421–3.

12. Kubler AC, Speder B, Zoller JE. Fronto-orbital advancement with simultaneous LeFort III-distraction. J Craniomaxillofac Surg. 2004; 32: 291–5.

13. Arnaud E, Marchac D, Renier D. Quadruple internal distraction with early frontal-facial avancement for faciocraniodysostosis. Rev Stomatol Chir Maxillofac. 2004; 105: 13–8.

14. Bradley JP, Gabbay JS, Taub PJ, et al. Monobloc advancement by distraction osteogenesis decreases morbidity and relapse. Plast Reconstr Surg. 2006; 118: 1585–97.

15. Joos U. Functional treatment of craniosynostoses during childhood. Br J Oral Maxillofac Surg. 1998; 36: 91–8.

16. Kumar AR, Steinbacher D. Advances in the treatment of syndromic midface hypoplasia using monobloc and facial bipartition distraction osteogenesis. Semin Plast Surg. 2014; 28: 179–83.

17. Taylor JA, Bartlett SP. What's New in syndromic craniosynostosis surgery? Plast Reconstr Surg. 2017; 140: 82e–93e.

18. Bradley JP, Levitt A, Nguyen J, et al. Roman arch, keystone fixation for facial bipartition with monobloc distraction. Plast Reconstr Surg. 2008; 122: 1514–23.

19. Kawamoto HK, Heller JB, Heller MM, et al. Craniofrontonasal dysplasia: a surgical treatment algorithm. Plast Reconstr Surg. 2007; 120: 1943–56.

20. Pinzer T, Gollogly J, Krishnan KG, Schackert G, Lauer G. Telecanthus and hypertelorism in frontoethmoidal meningoencephaloceles and the surgical correction of these conditions: Part II. A novel surgical approach in the treatment of telecanthus. J Craniofac Surg. 2008; 19: 148–55.

21. Jeelani NU, Khan MA, Fitzgerald O'Connor EJ, Dunaway D, Hayward R. Frontofacial monobloc distraction using the StealthStation intraoperative navigation system: the ability to see where you are cutting. J Craniofac Surg. 2009; 20: 892–4.

22. Adolphs N, Haberl EJ, Liu W, et al. Virtual planning for craniomaxillofacial surgery–7 years of experience. J Craniomaxillofac Surg. 2014; 42: e289–95.

23. Li D, Bai S, Yu Z, et al. Surgery navigation in treating congenital midfacial dysplasia of patients with facial cleft. J Craniofac Surg. 2017; 28: 1492–4.

CHAPTER 21

Posterior Skull Surgery in Craniosynostosis

Sgouros S, Goldin JH, Hockley AD, Wake MJC.
Child's Nerv Syst. 1996; 12: 727–33.

Reviewed by Neil J Opie

Research Question/Objective

The surgical management of raised intracranial pressure and abnormal head shape in craniosynostosis has focused on interventions that increase the cranial vault volume to allow the brain space to develop. Historically, procedures that addressed the anterior part of the skull (such a fronto-orbital advancement and remodelling) were utilised predominantly.

This paper describes the early experiences with posterior skull surgery by the Craniofacial Surgery Unit, Queen Elizabeth and Children's Hospitals, Birmingham, UK. This work subsequently laid the foundations for contemporary treatment approaches to complex craniosynostosis which have been adopted internationally by many units.

Study Design

The authors conducted a retrospective cohort study of children with craniosynostosis between 1978 and 1994.

Operative treatment was undertaken in 275 children with craniosynostosis during the study period. Of these, 22 had posterior skull surgery at some stage in their management (8%).

The 22 patients were divided into three groups:

I. Syndromic patients with complex multiple suture involvement (n = 16)
II. Non-syndromic patients with coronal and lambdoid suture involvement (n = 3)
III. Isolated lambdoid synostosis (n = 3)

All patients were assessed preoperatively with plain skull radiographs and three-dimensional computed tomography (3D CT) scans.

Postoperative follow-up included clinical assessment and skull radiographs, and clinical photographs were obtained at 3, 6, and 12 months postoperatively.

Sample Size

Twenty-two children (13 male) had posterior skull release surgery during the study period. This procedure was the primary operation in 13 cases.

Follow-up

Mean follow-up was 5.4 years (range: 1.5–12.5 years).

Inclusion/Exclusion Criteria

Inclusion criteria were any child who underwent posterior skull surgery as part of their craniosynostosis surgical management.

Intervention or Treatment Received

The methods employed to achieve posterior skull release were based on two main techniques:

    a. Circumferential-occipital craniectomy (Figure 21.1)
    b. Bilateral bone flap craniotomy (Figure 21.2)

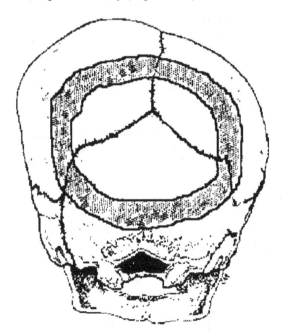

Figure 21.1   Circumferential-occipital craniectomy.

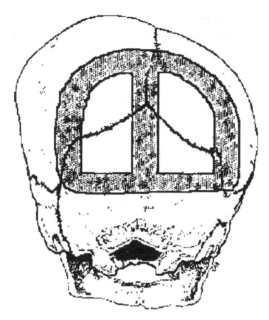

Figure 21.2 Bilateral bone flap craniotomy.

The circumferential occipital craniectomy was employed in all the syndromic patients (who invariably had bilateral lambdoid synostosis), with the bilateral flap technique utilised in non-syndromic patients.

Results

I. Syndromic complex craniosynostosis:

All 16 patients in this group had severe complex craniosynostosis involving both the anterior and the posterior suture complexes with radiological evidence of raised intracranial pressure.

Two male siblings presented successively with a variation of "clover-leaf" deformity, radiographic evidence of marked constriction in the posterior skull and significant "copper beating" predominantly in the occipital region. Both had early posterior skull surgery aged 6 weeks, and neither required further surgery. It was the excellent results obtained in these two cases that alerted the authors to the potential benefits of posterior skull release.

Seven further patients had early posterior skull surgery (mean age at operation: 4 months; range: 2.5–7 months). All skull radiographs revealed "copper beating," more marked posteriorly. Subsequently, fronto-orbital advancement procedures were performed after the age of 1 year (mean age at operation: 14.3 months; range: 3.5–24 months).

Three patients had early fronto-orbital advancement (2, 2, and 5 months, respectively). Significant residual "copper beating" in the occipital region on radiographs led to them undergoing posterior skull surgery 3 months later (5, 5 and 7 months of age respectively).

Four patients with complex craniosynostosis had posterior skull release as part of a series of transcranial operative procedures. The first of these was a patient with severe Crouzon syndrome who underwent posterior skull release at the age of 5 months. After this procedure, the patient's hydrocephalus progressed, which effectively achieved a frontal advancement by "pushing" the forehead forward. The hydrocephalus was treated with a ventriculo-peritoneal shunt. However, the patient retained a residual constriction at the midpart of the skull vault, which was then treated with a modified sagittal craniectomy 3 months later.

The second of these four patients had a ventriculo-peritoneal shunt for hydrocephalus, followed by posterior skull release at the age of 11 months. The hydrocephalus had again achieved frontal advancement in a similar fashion to the previous case. Although less severe, this patient also had a residual constriction in the mid-vault region, but it was felt that this did not merit surgical correction.

A third patient with Apert's syndrome had a calvarial morcellation procedure at the age of 5 months, followed by posterior skull release at 8 months and fronto-orbital advancement at 15 months.

A fourth patient with Antley-Bixler syndrome and hydrocephalus had a ventriculo-peritoneal shunt and posterior skull release at the age of 3 months, followed by bilateral temporal decompressive craniotomies 2 months later, and a fronto-orbital advancement at the age of 3 years.

II. Non-syndromic lambdoid and coronal synostosis:

Three patients with non-syndromic bilateral involvement of the lambdoid and coronal sutures had early posterior skull surgery (5, 5, and 6 months, respectively) for radiographic "copper beating" localised to the posterior skull, suggesting that the lambdoid synostosis was contributing to skull growth restriction.

The first two had subsequent fronto-orbital advancement (ages 14 and 16 months), while the third patient did not undergo additional surgery, as the head shape was considered satisfactory.

III. Isolated lambdoid synostosis:

Three patients with isolated lambdoid synostosis had posterior skull surgery (1% of all cases operated on for craniosynostosis in the study period). The ages of the patients at the time of surgery were 12, 14, and 15 months:

One had a good outcome with satisfactory remodelling of head shape and the other two patients had a degree of residual occipital deformity, but neither required further surgery.

The authors concluded that in patients with complex syndromes, posterior calvarial surgery relieves intracranial pressure and can improve head shape to the extent that fronto-orbital advancement may be unnecessary or can be delayed.

As a result of this case series, the Craniofacial Unit in Birmingham adopted a protocol whereby syndromic multiple-suture synostosis cases with radiographic evidence of "copper beating" and lambdoid synostosis causing restriction of skull growth posteriorly underwent posterior skull release in the first few months of life.

Study Limitations

This study comprised a relatively small sample size of 22 patients who underwent posterior skull surgery. The sample itself was heterogenous and variable; the patients who underwent the same surgery did not have similar baseline characteristics, nor did they all undergo the same procedures, at the same age, for the same indications.

Longer follow-up would have been preferable (minimum 10 years), and complex syndromic craniosynostosis patients would typically be expected to be followed up into adulthood.

While outcomes are recorded as "satisfactory" or "reasonable", no standardised objective measures are offered, nor is it clear what the significance of these patients not undergoing these procedures would have been.

Relevant Studies

Reoperation rates following fronto-orbital advancement have been reported in up to 100% in Apert patients, 65% in patients with Saethre–Chotzen syndrome, 38% in Pfeiffer, and 26% in Crouzon syndromes.[1]

The inadequacy of fronto-orbital advancement as the primary treatment modality for complex craniosynostosis patients is believed to be due to the relatively small gains in intracranial volume achieved with these procedures when compared to procedures on the posterior skull. Choi et al. found that when performing volumetric analysis of computer-simulated surgery, posterior cranial procedures were able to achieve approximately 35% greater intracranial volume expansions when compared to equivalent anterior cranial vault advancements.[2]

Procedures for expansion of the posterior cranial vault were developed to increase intracranial volume, address intracranial hypertension, and redirect cerebral expansion posteriorly. Initial techniques entailed formal cranioplasty with fixation of bone segments.[3,4,5]

Sgouros et al. described posterior skull surgery, which resulted in a free-floating occipital release.[6] These operative techniques exploit "brain drive" in infants to create posterior cranial vault expansion. Posteriorly directed brain growth and expansion is used to drive gradual displacement of the free-floating occipital bone, so that intracranial volume is increased and normalisation of head shape occurs.

One advantage of the technique described is the relatively minimal surgical manipulation required, thereby reducing the risk of dural tear. However, supine positioning in the postoperative period may prevent posterior expansion and could even potentially cause brain compression, resulting in relapse.[7]

Subsequent to the Sgouros paper, springs and internal distractors have been developed to expand the posterior skull.[8,9] White et al. were the first to describe posterior cranial distraction in 2009, this work having also been undertaken in the Birmingham Craniofacial Unit. Since then, other groups have adopted this approach internationally, and many units now consider posterior calvarial distraction the first line approach where significant vault expansion is required.[10–18]

There is still a place for the free-floating occipital release as described in the Sgouros paper. In young infants below 6 months of age with evidence of raised intracranial pressure, and where bone stock would not permit the use of distractors or springs, this technique may still "buy time" while the infant still retains the ability to regrow bone.

REFERENCES

1. Wong GB, Kakulis EG, Mulliken JB. Analysis of fronto-orbital advancement for, Crouzon, Pfeiffer, and Saethre–Chotzen syndromes. Plast Reconstr Surg. 2000; 105: 2314–23.
2. Choi M, Flores RL, Havlik RJ. Volumetric analysis of anterior versus posterior cranial vault expansion in patients with syndromic craniosynostosis. J Craniofac Surg. 2012; 23: 455–8.
3. Cinalli G, Chumas P, Arnaud E, Sainte-Rose C, Renier D. Occipital remodeling and suboccipital decompression in severe craniosynostosis associated with tonsillar herniation. Neurosurgery. 1998; 42: 66–71.
4. Persing JA, Jane JA, Delashaw JB. Treatment of bilateral coronal synostosis in infancy: a holistic approach. J Neurosurg. 1990; 72: 171–5.
5. Pollack IF, Losken HW, Hurwitz DJ. A combined frontoorbital and occipital advancement technique for use in total calvarial reconstruction. J Neurosurg. 1996; 84: 424–9.
6. Sgouros S, Goldin JH, Hockley AD, Wake MJ. Posterior skull surgery in craniosynostosis. Childs Nerv Syst. 1996; 12: 727–33.
7. Nowinski D, Di Rocco F, Renier D, et al. Posterior cranial vault expansion in the treatment of craniosynostosis. Comparison of current techniques. Child's Nervous System. 2012; 28: 1537–44.
8. Davis C, MacFarlane MR, Wickremesekera A. Occipital expansion without osteotomies in apert syndrome. Childs Nerv Syst. 2010; 26: 1543–8.

9. White N, Evans M, Dover MS, et al. Posterior calvarial vault expansion using distraction osteogenesis. Childs Nerv Syst. 2009; 25: 231-6.

10. Opie N, Evans M. Posterior calvarial osseodistraction for syndromic craniosynostosis. In Idle M and Monaghan A. (Eds.): Challenging Concepts in Oral and Maxillofacial Surgery. Oxford: Oxford University Press, 2016.

11. Nowinski D, Saiepour D, Leikola J, et al. Posterior cranial vault expansion performed with rapid distraction and time-reduced consolidation in infants with syndromic craniosynostosis. Childs Nerv Syst. 2011; 27: 1999-2003.

12. Serlo WS, Ylikontiola LP, Lahdesluoma N, et al. Posterior cranial vault distraction osteogenesis in craniosynostosis: estimated increases in intracranial volume. Childs Nerv Syst. 2011; 27: 627-33.

13. Steinbacher DM, Skirpan J, Puchala J, Bartlett SP. Expansion of the posterior cranial vault using distraction osteogenesis. Plast Reconstr Surg. 2011; 127: 792-801.

14. Thomas GP, Wall SA, Johnson D, et al. Lessons learned in posterior cranial vault distraction. J Craniofac Surg. 2014; 25: 1721-27.

15. Ylikontiola LP, Sandor GK, Salokorpi N, Serlo WS. Experience with craniosynostosis treatment using posterior calvarial distraction osteogenesis. Ann Maxillofac Surg. 2012; 2: 4-7.

16. Derderian CA, Bastidas N, Bartlett SP. Posterior cranial vault expansion with distraction osteogenesis, Childs Nerv Syst. 2012; 28: 1551-6.

17. Taylor JA, Derderian CA, Bartlett SP, et al. Perioperative morbidity in posterior cranial vault expansion: distraction osteogenesis versus conventional osteotomy. Plast Reconstr Surg. 2012; 129: 674e-80e.

CHAPTER 22

The Diagnosis and Management of Recurrent Aphthous Stomatitis: A Consensus Approach

Scully C, Gorsky M, Lozada-Nur F. J Am Dent Assoc. 2003; 134: 200–7.

Reviewed by Kathleen Fan and Emma Hayes

Research Question/Objective

Provide an update on the diagnosis and management of recurrent aphthous stomatitis (RAS).

Study Design

A collaborative approach to diagnosis and management of RAS based on expert experience and a review of the literature. The literature search was for papers published between 1995 and 2000 identified using a Medline search; however, the paper was not intended as a systematic review.

Study Limitations

No search strategy was used beyond the date range; it is a consensus approach by experts in the field of oral medicine.

It is worth noting that the papers included were on RAS and not oral ulceration secondary to other causes. Although the diagnosis of RAS is discussed, it was beyond the scope of the article to discuss the features of all other conditions associated with recurrent oral ulceration; therefore, the onus was placed on the clinician to ensure that they can distinguish RAS from ulceration related to systemic conditions. A useful overview of causes of oral ulceration is found in the review by Felix et al.[1] and although not an exhaustive list, a useful table of some associated features of recurrent oral ulceration can be found in the paper by Hullah.[2]

Study Findings

This paper builds upon the work of earlier papers, such as those by Scully and Porter,[3] published in 1989, covering the aetiology, pathogenesis, and management of RAS. Although many papers have been published since 1989, the description of the clinical features of minor, major, and herpetiform RAS described in this paper remain a useful and eloquent description. This can be easily visualised in the table in the later paper by Porter et al.[4] which highlights the differences between minor RAS, major RAS, and herpetiform RAS.

Distinguishing features of minor RAS included in the paper were a smaller number of ulcers per crop (1–5), smaller size (<10 mm), and healing without scarring within 2 weeks. Major RAS typically has larger ulcers (>10 mm), lasting over 30 days, and scarring is common. In addition, these ulcers can be found on the pharynx and palate, where they are not commonly found in minor RAS. Herpetiform ulcers have a different pattern, with multiple (10–100) small ulcers (1–2 mm), which may coalesce to form a larger ulcer; the age of onset is typically around 20–29 years.

A genetic basis for RAS was suggested, and precipitating factors included trauma, stress, foods, hormonal imbalance, and tobacco smoking.

The pathogenesis of RAS is thought to be related to a cell-mediated immune response with tumour necrosis factor α playing a major role.

A mononuclear cell infiltrate is thought to infiltrate the epithelium leading to papular swelling surrounded by vasculitic erythema. This papule ulcerates and a fibrinous membrane covers the ulcer. Finally, healing occurs by epithelial regeneration.

Diagnosis is made on the basis of the history and clinical findings, as there are no specific diagnostic tests.

The management of RAS is focused on reducing symptoms and discomfort, ulcer number and size, and increasing disease free periods. To help determine management strategies, the paper divided the clinical presentation of RAS into three types: A, B and C, and suggested strategies for each (although it should be noted that this is not a widely used convention).

Type A presentations are for relatively few days and only occur infrequently throughout the year, and management is based on trying to identify triggers and avoid them rather than medical treatment.

Type B represents painful ulcers that occur regularly every month, lasting 3–10 days. Preventative strategies are important, as are the identification of prodromal symptoms and early use of corticosteroids when present. Usually, short courses of corticosteroid mouthwash are sufficient, but a maintenance protocol may be required due to the consistent recurring pattern of the condition.

Type C indicates a chronic course whereby new ulcers develop before others have healed. Such patients should be treated by an oral medicine specialist and may require potent topical corticosteroids, systemic corticosteroids, or other potent immunosuppressant medications, including thalidomide.

Relevant Studies

There are many papers available on RAS, but as the exact aetiology remains unknown, curative treatment currently remains elusive. The variable nature of the condition, in terms of frequency of attacks, size, and the discomfort associated with ulceration, remains a challenge in producing good quality evidence and randomised controlled trials (RCTs). However, scoring systems such as that suggested by Tappuni et al.[5] which can be used easily on clinic as well as in trials, may improve the quality of data collection in the future.

A 2012 Cochrane review[6] summarises the available evidence for treatment of RAS in RCTs (with reduction in pain, frequency, or duration of ulceration as the outcome measures). Twenty-five trials were included, but "no single treatment was found to be effective and therefore the results remain inconclusive in regard to the best systemic intervention for RAS." Although some studies had statistically significant results, these were not considered to be sufficient to recommend use of systemic therapy due to the risk of bias in the study design or methodology.

The lack of RCT level data means that treatment for RAS is often guided by case reports, case series, and clinical experience. The case series by Lynde et al.[7] is notable for using a treatment ladder, which starts with colchicine (which is often used as a first-line agent for RAS if topical treatment is not sufficient), then adds dapsone for patients who do not respond. Although both colchicine and dapsone are used by oral medicine specialists, this paper shows that the combination increases the response rate to 80%. Patients were given 12 weeks to respond to colchicine before dapsone was added, and while treatment may be successful, response is not necessarily rapid. In addition, only those defined as having complex RAS were included. At present there is no study that has assessed if similar response rates are seen in patients who heal without scarring.

Many patients do not require systemic treatment. For all newly diagnosed patients, an underlying hematological deficiency should be excluded. The 1975 paper by Wray et al.[8] highlighted the association between B12, folate, and iron deficiencies in patient with RAS, with 17.7% of patients with RAS having a deficiency, compared to 8.5% of controls. In addition, those with deficiencies responded better to treatment when the deficiencies were managed compared to those without deficiencies. Further studies have found an increased frequency of hematological deficiencies in patients with RAS in different countries.[9,10]

Topical treatment remains the first line of therapy for RAS, and is used in addition to systemic medication, but there is no conclusive evidence regarding which topical therapies are effective. A consensus view in the literature is that treatment should start with elimination of precipitating factors, and the use of chlorhexidine, and protective or barrier treatments in both adults and children.[3,11,12] This is usually followed by topical corticosteroids in increasing levels of potency. The choice of topical corticosteroid depends not only on the diagnosis but also on the patient acceptability,[13] as well as drug availability, and therefore it is not possible to give a prescriptive list of which to use.

Topical corticosteroids available in the United Kingdom to use as a mouthwash (when dissolved in water) include betamethasone tablets, soluble prednisolone, and fluticasone capsules, which are relatively easy to use and cover large areas of the mucosa. For more localised treatment corticosteroids designed for nasal use (e.g., fluticasone aqueous spray) or asthma can be applied to a single ulcer. Alternatively, topical treatment can be in the form of steroid-based creams or ointments, of which a range of potencies is available, although the use of these may be limited by the dexterity required for application and acceptability to patients. A useful summary of the topical corticosteroids commonly used in oral medicine was written by Rudralingam et al.[13] Nearly all topical corticosteroids used in the mouth are used off-license, and therefore it is important that the prescriber understands the rationale and risks of their use.

The systematic review by Staines and Greenwood[14] highlights the inconclusive nature of the available evidence for topical therapies and states that this may be a reflection of the multifactorial nature of RAS in addition to study design or lack of appropriate studies. However, it found that when compared to placebo, the use of topical corticosteroids may be more effective in reducing pain and the duration of ulcers. The paucity of good quality RCTs on topical corticosteroid means that it is not possible to recommend one preparation over another.

REFERENCES

1. Felix DH, Luker J, Scully C. Oral medicine: 1. Ulcers: aphthous and other common ulcers. Dent Update. 2012; 39: 513–9.
2. Hullah EA. Oral ulceration: aetiology, diagnosis and treatment. Dental Nursing. 2014; 10: 507–12.
3. Scully C, Porter S. Recurrent aphthous stomatitis: current concepts of etiology, pathogenesis and management. J Oral Pathology Med. 1989; 18: 21–7.
4. Porter SR, Scully C, Pedersen A. Recurrent aphthous stomatitis. Crit Rev Oral Biol Med. 1998; 9: 306–21.
5. Tappuni AR, Kovacevic T, Shirlaw PJ, Challacombe SJ. Clinical assessment of disease severity in recurrent aphthous stomatitis. J Oral Pathol Med. 2013; 42: 635–41.
6. Brocklehurst P, Tickle M, Glenny AM, et al. Systemic interventions for recurrent aphthous stomatitis (mouth ulcers). Cochrane Database Syst Rev. 2012, (9). Art. No.: CD005411.

7. Lynde CB, Bruce AJ, Rogers RS. Successful treatment of complex aphthosis with colchicine and dapsone. Arch Dermatol. 2009; 145: 273–6.

8. Wray D, Ferguson MM, Mason DK, Hutcheon AW, Dagg JH. Recurrent aphthae: treatment with vitamin B12, folic acid, and iron. Br Med J. 1975; 2: 490–3.

9. Rogers RS III, Hutton KP. Screening for haematinic deficiencies in patients with recurrent aphthous stomatitis. Australas J Dermatol. 1986; 27: 98–103.

10. Khan NF, Saeed M, Chaudhary S, Khan NF. Haematological parameters and recurrent aphthous stomatitis. J Coll Physicians Surg Pak. 2013; 23: 124–7.

11. Woo SB, Sonis ST. Recurrent aphthous ulcers: a review of diagnosis and treatment. J Am Dent Assoc. 1996; 127: 1202–13.

12. Montgomery-Cranny JA, Wallace A, Rogers HJ, et al. Management of recurrent aphthous stomatitis in children. Dent Update. 2015; 42: 564–72.

13. Rudralingam M, Randall C, Mighell AJ. The use of topical steroid preparations in oral medicine in the UK. Br Dent J. 2017; 223: 633–8.

14. Staines K, Greenwood M. Aphthous ulcers (recurrent). Br Med J Clin Evid. 2015: 1303.

CHAPTER 23

Update on Oral Lichen Planus: Etiopathogenesis and Management

Scully C, Beyli M, Ferreiro MC, et al. Crit Rev Oral Biol Med. 1998; 9: 86–122.

Reviewed by Cameron M Herbert and Esther A Hullah

Research Question/Objective

A review article published by clinicians and scientists who are considered experts in the field of oral lichen planus (OLP). It was written following a European workshop in 1995 and aimed to highlight the challenges from an epidemiological, diagnostic, and management perspective.

Epidemiology

OLP has a high incidence in the general population (up to 4%) and often has characteristic features but may present in a number of different forms. The incidence increases from middle-age, and the female to male ratio is 2:1.

Clinical Presentation

The most common presentation is reticular white striae of the buccal mucosa, or tongue. Other forms such as plaques, ulceration and bullae may appear simultaneously or exclusively.

Pain is most commonly associated with erosions or ulceration.

Diagnosis of OLP is aided with histology and immunofluorescence to exclude conditions such as malignancy or vesiculo-bullous disorders. Histological features include hyperkeratosis, degenerative changes to the basal cells with a band-life infiltrate of lymphocytes and histocytes. Other features include the presence of colloid bodies, which have undergone premature keratinisation and have been extruded into the underlying mesenchyme. Plasma cells and macrophages may also be noted.

On histopathology, lichenoid reaction and lichen planus appear similar, making definitive diagnosis difficult without clinical correlation. Lichenoid reactions can be allergic in nature or reactions to toxic compounds. Histology can be helpful in the diagnosis of a drug-induced lichenoid reaction due to the increase in diffuse lymphocytic infiltrate, presence of eosinophils, plasma cells and an increase in colloid bodies.

Aetiology

The condition has a multifactorial etiopathogenesis and complex interactions. T-lymphocyte-mediated immunity has a major role in the pathogenesis of OLP. It is likely that external factors and patient's genetics contribute to the predisposition of developing OLP.

There has been suggested to be an association between autoimmune disease and OLP, but this is not clearly proven.[1] Hyperthyroidism, pemphigus vulgaris and Sjögren's syndrome are among the autoimmune conditions associated with the presentation of OLP.

Lichenoid reactions from dental materials have been reported with several studies, suggesting a proportion of patients with OLP demonstrate mercury sensitivity on patch-testing and removing amalgam restorations can provide improvement in some cases.[2] Composite restorations have however also been implicated in lichenoid reactions, and therefore replacing amalgam restorations with composite may not be warranted.

The literature reports lichenoid reactions in association with many common systemic therapies. Non-steroidal anti-inflammatory drugs and angiotensin-converting enzyme inhibitors are among those with the strongest associations. Other commonly prescribed classes associated include thiazide diuretics, penicillamine, beta-blockers, quinine and quinidine, para-amino salicylic acid, phenothiazines, carbamazepine, allopurinol, lithium, lorazepam, ketoconazole, streptomycin, isoniazid, metopromazine, levopromazine, amiphenazole, pyrimethamine, levamisole, beta-blocking agents, cinnarizine, flunarizine, gold and cyanamide. Treatment of drug reaction lichenoid reactions includes removal of the causative agent; however, patients' systemic conditions may be more life-threatening than the lichenoid reaction itself.

Infectious agents have long been noted in the context of OLP; however, their causative role remains undetermined. A relationship with gram-negative anaerobic bacilli has been suggested but not proven. Lichenoid lesions have been reported in relation to syphilitic chronic bladder infections and intestinal amebiasis, and improvements have been noted when treated with metronidazole.

Candida albicans has been found in OLP on mycology and histological studies, and treatment with anti-fungal therapy can sometimes improve OLP. Viruses have been implicated in OLP, including human immunodeficiency virus, human papilloma virus, and Epstein-Barr virus. Lichen planus has been diagnosed in 5% of patients with hepatitis C (HCV) infection, and treatment of HCV with interferon may improve OLP.[3]

A number of patients with lichenoid lesions have been noted to have a reaction to food additives such as cinnamon-aldehyde.

Malignant Potential

The potential of malignant transformation of OLP and lichenoid reactions has long been debated and it considered to occur in approximately 1%, with smoking, alcohol, and chronic liver disease being contributing factors.[4]

Given the premalignant potential of OLP, it is recommended that patients should be reviewed on a regular basis. Patients should be advised on how to monitor and contact their health-care provider should they notice any change to their OLP.

Treatment

The effects of OLP on quality of life depend largely on the clinical type, with ulcerative and erosive being the most uncomfortable.

Lichen planus that is nonerosive and nonsymptomatic does not require active treatment. The presentations of erosive, ulcerated, and atrophic lichen planus often lead to difficulty in patients maintaining adequate oral hygiene, and toothbrushing can be particularly uncomfortable, with resulting problematic gingival bleeding. Good oral hygiene practices may produce subjective and objective improvement of oral lichen planus lesions.

Localised areas of mechanical trauma should be addressed, as these are known to result in the Köebner's phenomenon, a common feature in OLP.

Immunomodulatory drugs, particularly steroid-based therapies, provide the mainstay for treatment of OLP.

Systemic corticosteroids such as prednisolone can successfully control OLP; however, adverse effects from systemic steroid therapy are seen even with short courses of just 2 weeks, and therefore they are generally reserved for cases resistant to local measures.[5] Greater symptom control has actually been demonstrated with topical corticosteroids.

Betamethasone pellets used as a mouthwash, topical clobetasol and fluocinonide have been demonstrated to be helpful in treating OLP, with no evidence that one preparation is better than others.[5]

Intra-lesional steroid treatment is effective at healing for localised erosive lesions only.

Where steroid therapy is not effective, other immunomodulatory drugs are suggested including topical cyclosporin, tacrolimus, and thalidomide.[6] Systemic

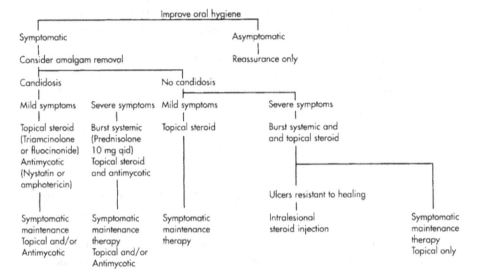

Figure 23.1   Algorithm for the management of area lichen planus. (Adopted from Oliver and Winkelman 1993.) HE, hematoxylin and eosin; PAS, periodic-acid-Schiff.

steroid sparing agents such as azathioprine are also reported to have effect in OLP. Long-term systemic implications of such immunosuppressive therapy, including long-term malignancy risk, should be considered.

Other proposed therapies include photodynamic therapy and low-level laser therapy.[6]

Patients on corticosteroid or immunomodulation therapies for the treatment of their OLP are more predisposed to candida overgrowth which can in turn worsen their OLP symptoms. It has been demonstrated that reducing the candida burden can reduce erosive lesions to reticular level lesions.

An algorithm is provided to guide the clinical management of OLP and is still applicable today (Figure 23.1).

Paper Limitations

More recent papers are available reviewing OLP, including the use of newer systemic pharmacological agents which therefore limit the usefulness of this review. A recent review of the up-to-date OLP literature reports the aetiology of lichen planus remains unknown.[7] It discusses the modified WHO diagnostic criteria of OLP and oral lichenoid lesions, which has been updated since the publication of the review paper. Similar findings were also noted by another review, which reports a correlation between HCV infection and OLP.[8] There has been little in the way of evidence for novel therapies which may be beneficial in control of OLP.

REFERENCES

1. López-Jornet P, Parra-Perez F, Pons-Fuster A. Association of autoimmune diseases with oral lichen planus: a cross-sectional, clinical study. J Eur Acad Dermatol Venereol. 2014; 28: 895–9.
2. Thornhill MH, Pemberton MN, Simmons RK, Theaker ED. Amalgam-contact hypersensitivity lesions and oral lichen planus. Oral Surg Oral Med Oral Pathol Oral Radiol Endod. 2003; 95: 291–9.
3. Nagao Y, Sata M. A retrospective case-control study of hepatitis C virus infection and oral lichen planus in Japan: association study with mutations in the core and NS5A region of hepatitis C virus. BMC Gastroenterol. 2012; 12: 31.
4. Aghbari SM, Abushouk AI, Attia A, et al. Malignant transformation of oral lichen planus and oral lichenoid lesions: a meta-analysis of 20095 patient data. Oral Oncol. 2017; 68: 92–102.
5. Lodi G, Manfredi M, Mercadante V, Murphy R, Carrozzo M. Interventions for treating oral lichen planus: corticosteroid therapies. Cochrane Database Syst Rev. 2020; 2:CD001168.
6. Yang H, Wu Y, Ma H, et al. Possible alternative therapies for oral lichen planus cases refractory to steroid therapies. Oral Surg Oral Med Oral Pathol Oral Radiol. 2016; 121: 496–509.
7. Alrashdan MS, Cirillo N, McCullough M. Oral lichen planus: a literature review and update. Arch Dermatol Res. 2016; 308: 539–51.
8. Kurago ZB. Etiology and pathogenesis of oral lichen planus: an overview. Oral Surg Oral Med Oral Pathol Oral Radiol. 2016; 122: 72–80.

CHAPTER 24

The Radiological Prediction of Inferior Alveolar Nerve Injury during Third Molar Surgery

Rood JP, Shehab N. Br J Oral Maxillofac Surg. 1990; 28: 20–5.

Reviewed by Vinod Patel

Research Question/Objective

Inferior dental/alveolar nerve (IDN) injury (IDNI) is the most concerning complication associated with mandibular third molar (MTM) surgery (MTMS). These injuries are multi factorial. Radiological features are routinely used to assess the proximity and relationship of the MTM to the inferior alveolar canal (IAC), which is often regarded as the most significant factor. Two-dimensional imaging (e.g., orthopantomogram [OPG]) is the first investigation of choice, and is an integral part of the overall assessment. Historically, various permutations of radiological appearances of the IAC in relation to the MTM have been reported as being associated with IDNI. This study identified seven radiological signs repeatedly highlighted in the literature and assessed these against the risk of IDNI.

Study Design

This paper had two separate sub-studies both focusing on the same outcome of IDNI following MTMS in a population determined to be "at risk." This was based on seven pre-determined radiographic appearances established as risk factors for this complication. The two sub-studies were categorised as a case control (retrospective) and cohort (prospective). In both, the sample groups were collated over two centres providing MTMS. Cases were randomly selected for the retrospective group, but it is unclear if the same methodology was used for the prospective group. No blinding occurred in either study and both aimed to determine the presence of neurological deficit post-MTMS.

Sample Size

A total of 1,105 patients with 1,560 MTMs were included in this study. The sample size was split, with the retrospective group including 553 patients (800 MTMs) and the prospective group including 552 patients (760 MTMs).

Follow-up

IDNI for each patient in the retrospective study was identified via medical records. In comparison, in the prospective study patients were examined on the first postoperative day and again at a follow-up appointment, 7–10 days later. Neurological sensation was assessed using cotton wool, blunt probe, and a pinprick evaluation.

Inclusion/Exclusion Criteria

Patients requiring MTMS who presented with one or more of the predetermined radiological signs on two-dimensional imaging were included. The seven signs were (1) darkening of the root, (2) deflected roots, (3) narrowing of the root, (4) dark and bifid root, (5) interruptions of the white line(s), (6) diversion of the IAC and (7) narrowing of the IAC. Patients with isolated submental anesthesia without involvement of the lower lip or gingivae post-surgery were excluded.

Intervention or Treatment Received

All patients in both groups underwent complete removal of the MTM.

Results

Details of patient demographics were not given. The experience of the surgeons was also not described, but it was noted that clinicians with varying degree of skill undertook the procedures. Only the radiographic findings of the MTM were categorised, and this was based on the seven radiographic signs in the inclusion criteria.

A total of five signs (interruption of the white lines, darkening of the root, deflection of the root, diversion of the IAC ($p < 0.001$), and narrowing of the root ($p < 0.01$) were found to be statistically significantly associated with IDNI in the retrospective group. In the prospective study, only three signs (interruption of the white lines, darkening of the root, diversion of the IAC) ($p < 0.001$) were statistically significantly associated with IDNI.

The authors hypothesised that the most significant signs for IDNI were the three identified in the prospective study. This hypothesis was further strengthened, as these signs were also significantly found in the retrospective study, suggesting consistency. However, the retrospective study incidence was 25 IDNIs for 73 "at risk" signs, whereas in the prospective study it was 21 IDNIs for 157 "at risk" signs with both groups having a similar number of patients and number of MTMs extracted.

Of the three signs identified, diversion of the IAC was deemed the most significant ($X^2 = 53.0027$) with the interpreted conclusion that one in three patients would suffer a nerve injury with this radiographic presentation.

Both darkening of the root ($X^2 = 33.4157$) and interruption of the white line ($X^2 = 13.9134$) were risk assessed as one in four patients being likely to suffer a nerve injury.

Narrowing and deflection of the root were only found to be significant in the retrospective study, and the authors suggested that these signs are indicators for IDNI rather than significant radiographic risk factors. Narrowing of the IAC and a dark/bifid apex were not significantly associated with IDNI in either study.

Study Limitations

In the retrospective study, the IDNI was determined from the medical records. It is not clear whether the routine clinical practice was to follow-up patients post-MTMS and whether true capture of all IDNIs was achieved or whether this was based on patients' self-reporting. In contrast, for the prospective group all patients were followed up.

With regard to radiographic assessment, the study did not state whether one or multiple clinicians were involved in assessing them, leading to potential inter- and intra-observer error. The authors correctly highlighted that when multiple "at risk" signs are present, the risk of IDNI increases, but they were unable to stratify this risk due to small numbers. Additionally, it was recognised that twice as many "at risk" radiographic signs were identified in the prospective study cohort than in the retrospective cohort, most likely due to improved image quality of the panoramic radiographs and a larger proportion of cases having both periapical and OPG radiographs. There therefore remains a lack of consistency between these two studies, which is highly significant considering that the focus of this study is based around radiographic presentation.

Relevant Studies

This study continues to have significant relevance both in clinical practice and in the literature as two-dimensional imaging (OPG) is still the primary and routine imaging modality used to assess IDNI risk preoperatively.

This study highlights three radiographic signs: interruption of the IAC, deviation of the IAC, and darkening (banding) of the root as significant predictors for IDNI. Since the publication of this study, these radiographic signs have been scrutinised further following the introduction and increasing use of cone beam computed tomography (CBCT) in MTMS to assess such risk. CBCT imaging has been proven to provide good spatial and anatomical accuracy in identifying bucco-lingual position of the IAC and root morphology of the MTM,[1-4] but the additional value of this information does not appear to provide a clinical advantage with a reduction in IDNI as highlighted by numerous studies.[3,5,6]

When considering interruption of the IAC on 2D imaging, Nakagawa et al.[7] identified that only 86% of cases showed contact between the MTM roots and the IAC on CBCT and concluded an increasing risk of IDNI. This risk increases further with the increasing number of CBCT slices showing loss of integrity.[8] Darkening of the root or "banding" has traditionally been considered to be related to grooving of the root and loss of dental tissue and subsequently intimacy between them. However, CBCT review of this sign identified that in 80% of cases this was due to cortical thinning or perforation of the cortical plate[9] rather than the tooth root itself.

The assessment of MTMs deemed to be "at risk" of IDNI is often only considered in terms of the radiographic signs of the relationship between the tooth and the IAC. Nerve injuries are, however, multi factorial and other factors can be divided into three categories: surgical, tooth, and patient related.

Surgical factors include operator skill, with junior clinicians having a higher risk of IDNI.[10,11] Post-extraction exposure of the nerve is associated with IDNI.[12]

Tooth-related factors that are associated with IDNI include angle of impaction, with horizontal impactions considered highest risk, but this has not been consistently shown.[13-15] Increasing depth of impaction is associated with IDNI and is linked to eruption status, with unerupted teeth carrying a heightened risk.[13,14,16]

Finally, regarding patient factors, increasing age has been acknowledged as raising the risk of IDNI.[11,17,18]

None of these factors were considered in the paper presented and should not be overlooked, a fact highlighted in the study, as five patients were identified as having an IDNI post-MTMS without any of the "at risk" seven radiographic signs being present.

REFERENCES

1. Tantanapornkul W, Okouchi K, Fujiwara Y, et al. A comparative study of cone-beam computed tomography and conventional panoramic radiography in assessing the topographic relationship between the mandibular canal and impacted third molars. Oral Surg Oral Med Oral Pathol Oral Radiol Endod. 2007; 103: 253–9.
2. Ghaeminia H, Meijer GJ, Soehardi A, et al. Position of the impacted third molar in relation to the mandibular canal. Diagnostic accuracy of cone beam computed tomography compared with panoramic radiography. Int J Oral Maxillofac Surg. 2009; 38: 964–71.
3. Guerrero ME, Nackaerts O, Beinsberger J, et al. Inferior alveolar nerve sensory disturbance after impacted mandibular third molar evaluation using cone beam computed tomogra-phy and panoramic radiography: a pilot study. J Oral Maxillofac Surg. 2012; 70: 2264–70.

4. Hauge Matzen L, Christensen J, Hintze H, Schou S, Wenzel A. Diagnostic accuracy of panoramic radiography, stereo-scanography and cone beam CT for assessment of mandibular third molars before surgery. Acta Odontol Scand. 2013; 71: 1391–8.

5. Guerrero ME, Botetano R, Beltran J, Horner K, Jacobs R. Can preoperative imaging help to predict postoperative outcome after wisdom tooth removal? A randomized controlled trial using panoramic radiography versus cone-beam CT. Clin Oral Investig. 2013; 18: 335–42.

6. Suomalainen A, Apajalahti S, Vehmas T, Ventä I. Availability of CBCT and iatrogenic alveolar nerve injuries. Acta Odontol Scand. 2013; 71: 151–6.

7. Nakagawa Y, Ishii H, Nomura Y, et al. Third molar position: reliability of panoramic radiography. J Oral Maxillofac Surg. 2007; 65: 1303–8.

8. Park W, Choi JW, Kim JY, et al. Cortical integrity of the inferior alveolar canal as a predictor of paresthesia after third-molar extraction. J Am Dent Assoc. 2010; 141: 271–8.

9. Tantanapornkul W, Okochi K, Bhakdinaronk A, Ohbayashi N, Kurabayashi T. Correlation of darkening of impacted mandibular third molar root on digital panoramic images with cone beam computed tomography findings. Dentomaxillofac Radiol. 2009; 38: 11–6.

10. Jerjes W, Swinson B, Moles DR, et al. Permanent sensory nerve impairment following third molar surgery: a prospective study. Oral Surg Oral Med Oral Pathol Oral Radiol Endod. 2006; 102: e1–e7.

11. Cheung LK, Leung YY, Chow LK, et al. Incidence of neurosensory deficits and recovery after lower third molar surgery: a prospective clinical study of 4338 cases. Int J Oral Maxillofac Surg. 2010; 39: 320–6.

12. Bell GW. Use of dental panoramic tomographs to predict the relation between mandibular third molar teeth and the inferior alveolar nerve. Radiological and surgical findings, and clinical outcome. Br J Oral Maxillofac Surg. 2004; 42: 21–7.

13. Kipp DP, Goldstein BH, Weiss WW Jr. Dysesthesia after mandibular third molar surgery: a retrospective study and analysis of 1,377 surgical procedures. J Am Dent Assoc. 1980; 100: 185–92.

14. Carmichael FA, McGowan DA. Incidence of nerve damage following third molar removal: a West of Scotland Oral Surgery Research Group study. Br J Oral Maxillofac Surg. 1992; 30: 78–82.

15. Visintini E, Angerame D, Costantinides F, Maglione M. Peripheral neurological damage following lower third molar removal. A preliminary clinical study. Minerva Stomatol. 2007; 56: 319–26.

16. Gulicher D, Gerlach KL. Sensory impairment of the lingual and inferior alveolar nerves following removal of impacted mandibular third molars. Int J Oral Maxillofac Surg. 2001; 30: 306–12.

17. Black CG. Sensory impairment following lower third molar surgery: a prospective study in New Zealand. N Z Dent J. 1997; 93: 68–71.

18. Bruce RA, Frederickson GC, Small GS. Age of patients and morbidity associated with mandibular third molar surgery. J Am Dent Assoc. 1980; 101: 240–5.

CHAPTER 25

Impacted Maxillary Canines: A Review

Bishara SE. Am J Orthod Dentofacial Orthop. 1992; 101: 159–71.

Reviewed by Alice Cameron and Serryth Colbert

Research Question/Objective

This paper presents an overview of the incidence and sequelae, as well as the surgical, periodontal, and orthodontic considerations in the management of impacted canines. However, it was not expressed as a clearly focused question and the population included was not been explicitly specified.

Study Design

A review of the literature.

Inclusion/Exclusion Criteria

Not stated. The authors did not detail which bibliographic medical databases were used, whether unpublished and published studies were included and if non-English language studies were also used; this causes difficulty in assessing whether all relevant studies were included in this paper.

Results

The incidence of maxillary canine impaction was found to be between 0.92% and 1.7% and was twice as common in females compared to males. Eighty-three percent of labially impacted canines were associated with an arch length deficiency; these may erupt spontaneously, whereas palatally impacted canines seldom erupted without intervention.

Causes of retarded eruption of teeth were described as generalised and localised, with no clear explanation in most cases for the failure of eruption of the canine, although this was associated with abnormalities in the formation and eruption of the lateral incisor.

Although in some cases there were no untoward effects of impacted maxillary canines, their potential sequelae included resorption of lateral incisor root, which can extend into the pulp, estimated as occurring in 0.6–0.8% of children in the 11–13 age group. Another potential sequela noted was dentigerous cyst formation, estimated as occurring in up to 9.5% of cases.

An accurate diagnosis relies on clinical examination supplemented by radiographic images, using a tube shift (parallax) technique with plain x-ray films, to locate the impacted canine.

While a variety of treatment options are available to recover impacted maxillary canines, understanding the aetiology of impaction can guide early intervention, reducing the frequency of subsequent impaction. Selective extraction of the deciduous canine before 11 years of age can normalise the position of the ectopically erupting permanent canine; success rates are dependent on the position of the permanent canine crown in relation to the midline of the lateral incisor.

Treatment options included in this review were no active intervention, extraction of the ectopic canine (followed by auto-transplantation of the canine, movement of a first premolar into its position, posterior segmental osteotomy to medialise the buccal segment to close the space) or surgical exposure of the canine and orthodontic treatment to align. The deciduous canine is unlikely to survive forever, and this should be factored into treatment planning.

Where no treatment is planned, regular clinical and radiographic review is recommended to monitor for any pathological changes.

Natural eruption may follow surgical exposure, or auxiliary attachments can apply orthodontic force. Different forms of orthodontic traction may be applied including fixed and removable appliances. Only enough bone should be removed to enable visualisation of the crown, as increased bone removal is noted to reduce later alveolar bone support. The auxiliary attachment may be placed immediately or following placement of a healing dressing, with the latter suggested to allow more favourable placement of the attachment and vector control. Apically repositioned flaps are recommended for labially placed canines to ensure there is keratinised mucosa at the cementoenamel junction to optimise periodontal health and minimise recession.

Current practice continues to recognise the importance of maintaining maxillary canines, as the absence of one or more of these teeth may give rise to functional and aesthetic difficulties.[1] Extraction should only be considered in the presence of resorption of the canine or adjacent incisors, significant abnormality of morphology (e.g., dilaceration), position, or ankylosis where its retention would interfere with the health or orthodontic movement of other teeth.

Study Limitations

It is difficult to assess whether the authors included all relevant and important studies due to the lack of information regarding their inclusion and exclusion criteria and search techniques. There was little to indicate they had considered the rigor of the studies identified, though the reference list was lengthy and contained both clinical and radiographic studies, some of which continue to provide the evidence base for the treatment of impacted maxillary canines.

The use of conventional plain film radiography was discussed, notably the need for a second plain film image concomitantly with a tube-shift technique. This paper only briefly discussed the use of more elaborate radiographic techniques, such as polytomography, and this was only in relation to the sensitivity of diagnosis of resorption of the lateral incisor root and not regarding the localisation of impacted maxillary canines.

The two main drawbacks of conventional radiography in parallax techniques remain unchanged: anatomical superimposition and geometric distortion, both of which may ultimately affect the accurate localisation and therefore treatment planning of impacted canines. It should be recognised that other imaging modalities, such as cone beam computed tomography (CBCT), are now more frequently used to inform treatment planning in the localisation of impacted maxillary canines and overcome the aforementioned drawbacks of conventional parallax technique. In current practice, the most common means of radiographic localisation are through parallax and CBCT.[4] Furthermore, CBCT increases the detection of resorption associated with unerupted teeth by 50%.[2]

Interceptive treatment remains a feature of today's practice, and the authors documented percentage successes of normalising the position of the ectopically erupting permanent canine, which varied depending on the position of its crown, in patients before the age of 11 years. There was no comment with regard to success rates of the same in patients older than 11 years.

Some techniques described in this paper are no longer routinely performed, either because they had a weak evidence base or have been superseded by techniques with a more rigorous evidence base. This paper discusses surgical exposure to allow natural eruption to occur and the placement of a polycarboxylate crown onto the impacted tooth, post-exposure. This is infrequently carried out in current practice and has been replaced with techniques such as apically repositioned flaps or open exposure. Similarly, a two-step approach is discussed for the surgical exposure and placement of an auxiliary attachment, where the canine is surgically uncovered and immediately packed with a surgical dressing. Pack removal occurs after 3–8 weeks when the attachment was placed.[3]

An aspect of impacted maxillary canines which is highly relevant to our current clinical practice and one which was likely to have been less of an issue at the time of this paper's publication is that late or failed diagnosis, with subsequent resorption of an adjacent lateral incisor root. This is a potentially significant source of litigation for the general dental practitioner, orthodontic specialist, or oral and maxillofacial surgeon.

Overall results are not demonstrated in terms of number needed to treat (NNT), odds ratio, or other statistical analyses. When combined with more up-to-date, high-quality evidence-based literature, this paper still forms the basis of our diagnosis of and management for impacted maxillary canines. Diagnostic techniques have progressed and refined, while surgical techniques have favoured possibly more minimally invasive approaches, i.e., radical bone removal and the use of heavy exposure have been superseded.

Relevant Studies

Eslami et al.[4] outlined that CBCT is more effective than conventional radiography in evaluating cases that are difficult to diagnose during initial assessment with conventional radiography. The accuracy of CBCT ranged from 50% to 95%, while the accuracy of conventional radiography ranged from 39% to 85%. Without robust evidence to support CBCT use as a first-line choice of imaging for impacted maxillary canine evaluation, it is currently only indicated when conventional radiography does not provide adequate diagnostic information.[4]

A more robust evidence base for prognostic factors, used as an index to estimate treatment difficulty in assessing maxillary canines for interceptive management, has been developed. Four aspects of canine position should be assessed, and the patient's age considered. These prognostic factors are:

1. The amount of canine crown which horizontally overlaps the adjacent incisor
2. The vertical height of the canine crown
3. The canine angulation to the midline
4. The position of the canine root apex in the horizontal plane

Analysis of these factors allow prognosis for realignment to be categorised as good, average and poor, helping to inform treatment planning.[1]

The Royal College of Surgeons of England Faculty of Dental Surgery guidelines on *The Management of the Palatally Ectopic Maxillary Canine* recommend that less experienced practitioners should seek a specialist orthodontist opinion prior to initiating treatment.[5]

The results of several more recent studies have shown that the surgical exposure and orthodontic eruption of palatally impacted maxillary canines has minor effects on the periodontium.[3] Studies on open surgical exposure of impacted maxillary canines have shown minimal effects on the periodontium.[6]

In a randomised controlled trial, Parkin et al.[7] found no difference in surgical outcome between open and closed exposure of palatally displaced maxillary canines. Björksved et al. also undertook a randomised controlled trial comparing open and closed treatment for palatally impacted maxillary canines and found that there was no significant difference in surgical time or post-operative complications between the two groups, although those in the open group experienced more pain and impairment.[8]

REFERENCES

1. Counihan K, Al-Awadhi E, Butler J. Guidelines for the assessment of the impacted maxillary canine. Dent Update. 2013; 40: 770–7.
2. Ericsson S, Kurol J. Resorption of incisors after ectopic eruption of maxillary canines: a CT study. Angle Orthod. 2000; 70: 415–23.
3. Bedoya M, Park J. A review of the diagnosis and management of impacted maxillary canines. J Am Dent Assoc. 2009; 140: 1485–93.
4. Eslami E, Barkhordar H, Abramovitch K, Kim J, Masoud M. Cone-beam computed tomography vs conventional radiography in visualization of maxillary impacted-canine localization: a systematic review of comparative studies. Am J Orthodont Dentofac Orthoped. 2017; 151: 248–58.
5. Husain J, Burden D, McSherry P. Management of the palatally ectopic maxillary canine. *Royal College of Surgeons Faculty of Dental Surgery.* 2016. [Available from: https://www.rcseng.ac.uk/dental-faculties/fds/publications-guidelines/clinical-guidelines/.]
6. Schmidt A, Kokich V. Periodontal response to early uncovering, autonomous eruption, and orthodontic alignment of palatally impacted maxillary canines. Am J Orthodont Dentofac Orthoped. 2007; 131: 449–55.
7. Parkin NA, Deery C, Smith AM, et al. No difference in surgical outcomes between open and closed exposure of palatally displaced maxillary canines. J Oral Maxillofac Surg. 2012; 70: 2026–34.
8. Björksved M, Arnrup K, Lindsten R, et al. Closed vs open surgical exposure of palatally displaced canines: surgery time, postoperative complications, and patients' perceptions: a multicentre, randomized, controlled trial. Eur J Orthodont. 2018; 40: 626–35.

CHAPTER 26

Outcomes of Nonsurgical Retreatment and Endodontic Surgery: A Systematic Review

Torabinejad M, Corr R, Handysides R, Shabahang S.
J Endod. 2009; 35: 930–7.

Reviewed by Johno Breeze

Objective

To identify and compare papers describing the clinical and radiographic success rates of nonsurgical retreatment of root-filled teeth with those of teeth treated by surgical endodontics to determine which modality offers more favourable outcomes.[1]

Study Design

Systematic review and meta-analysis using the Patient Population, Intervention, Comparison, and Outcome (PICO) framework. Electronic databases were supplemented by the handpicking of journal articles from recognised endodontic journals.

Sample Size

Twenty-six endodontic surgery and eight nonsurgical retreatment articles were included. The publication date ranged from 1998 to 2008 for nonsurgical retreatment literature and from 1970 to 2008 for the endodontic surgery literature. A total of 8,198 teeth were included in the meta-analysis. Sample sizes within individual papers ranged from 27 to 1,016 teeth.

Follow-up

Follow-up periods within individual identified articles ranged between 6 months and 12 years.

Inclusion/Exclusion Criteria

Inclusion criteria for this review were articles from peer-reviewed journals published in English from 1970 to 2008 that reported clinical and/or radiographic outcomes data for nonsurgical endodontic retreatment or endodontic surgery. Inclusion criteria also included studies that reported follow-up data for a minimum of 25 teeth and a minimum 2-year mean follow-up period.

Surgical endodontics specifically describes a procedure combining root-end resection, apical curettage, and root-end filling. Other procedures such as apical curettage or root resection alone, hemisection, intentional replantation, and regenerative procedures have not been included.

Exclusion criteria consisted of studies that did not meet the above inclusion criteria, studies that reported outcomes based on individual roots as opposed to whole teeth, studies that did not report clinical or radiographic outcomes, animal studies, or studies that reported histologic data only.

Treatment Received

Nonsurgical retreatment of root-filled teeth versus those treated by surgical endodontics.

Results

A significantly higher success rate was found for endodontic surgery at 2–4 years (78%) compared with nonsurgical retreatment (71%). At 4–6 years, however, this relationship was reversed, with nonsurgical retreatment showing a higher success rate (83%) than surgery (72%).

Surgery had a significant decrease in success with each increasing follow-up interval. Weighted success at 2–4 years was 78%, 72% at 4–6 years and 63% at over 6 years. Conversely, the nonsurgical retreatment success rates demonstrated a statistically significant increase in weighted success from 2–4 years (71%) to 4–6 years (83%).

Study Limitations

Only one article meeting the criteria for inclusion made a direct comparison between endodontic surgery and nonsurgical retreatment.[2] Insufficient numbers of articles were available to make comparisons after 6 years of follow-up.

Relevant Studies

A wide range of success rates for initial root canal treatment have been reported.[1-4] Lack of healing is attributed to persistent intra-radicular infection residing in previously un-instrumented canals and dentinal tubules, or in the complex irregularities of the root canal system.[5] The extra-radicular causes of endodontic failures include periapical actinomycosis,[6] foreign body reaction caused by extruded endodontic material,[7] accumulation of endogenous cholesterol crystals in the apical tissues,[8] and an unresolved cystic lesion.[9]

The main options to manage previously root-treated teeth with persistent periapical lesions might be limited to nonsurgical retreatment or endodontic surgery, assuming the tooth is restorable and has sound periodontal health, and the patient wants to retain the tooth.[10] Nonsurgical retreatment may provide a better opportunity to clean the pulp space than a surgical approach.[11] However, there are clinical situations when nonsurgical root canal retreatment is inappropriate.[12]

The use of magnification during endodontic procedures, particularly using the dental operating microscope, provides enhanced visualisation of the operating field. Studies analysing the use of a microscope have shown high rates of success for both endodontic surgery[13] and nonsurgical retreatment.[14] Despite these benefits, the majority of articles in this systematic review did not report the use of magnification aids.

Studies that have made direct comparisons among root-end filling materials have consistently shown that modern materials such as mineral trioxide aggregate (MTA) offer more favourable clinical outcomes when compared with amalgam.[15] Three-quarters of articles in this systematic review, however, reported the use of amalgam as a root-end filling material. A meta-analysis of root-end filling materials by Fernandez-Yanez et al.[16] reported that amalgam is associated with the lowest success rate compared with intermediate restorative material (IRM), super ethoxybenzoic acid cement (Super-EBA), and MTA. They also noted that MTA was the most biocompatible material studied and offers the best physical properties in vitro.

In the United Kingdom, the Royal College of Surgeons of England indications for surgical endodontics[12] are widely used, based upon El-Swiah and Walker's paper.[17] These are:

1. Peri-radicular disease associated with a tooth where iatrogenic or developmental anomalies prevent nonsurgical root canal treatment being undertaken.
2. Peri-radicular disease in a root-filled tooth where nonsurgical root canal retreatment cannot be undertaken or has failed, or when it may be detrimental to the retention of the tooth.
3. Where a biopsy of peri-radicular tissue is required.
4. Where visualisation of the peri-radicular tissues and tooth root is required when perforation or root fracture is suspected.
5. Where it may not be expedient to undertake prolonged nonsurgical root canal retreatment because of patient considerations.

Two years before this systematic review was published, a Cochrane review by Del Fabbro et al. in 2007 had found similar results,[18] in that only two randomised controlled trials exist[2,11] that directly compared nonsurgical endodontic retreatment with endodontic surgery. Both articles had significant limitations. One was a study by Danin et al. in 1999,[11] who reported one-year postoperative follow-up data of only 38 patients. The small sample size and short follow-up time in this study are generally felt to be insufficient to adequately assess long-term success.[2] The other randomised study was by Kvist and Reit[2] on 95 teeth, finding better short-term outcomes for surgery, but no difference at 48 months.

The overall conclusion from the studies identified in this systematic review suggests that endodontic surgery offers more favourable initial success, but nonsurgical retreatment offers a more favourable long-term outcome, certainly over 48 months.

Where endodontic surgery has failed, repeating the periapical surgical procedure is associated with a significantly worse (59% compared to 86% completely healed radiographically) radiographic outcomes at 5 years.[19]

The long-term failure of endodontically treated and particularly endodontic surgery treated teeth has led some to question whether extraction and placement of a dental implant would have a better long-term prognosis, but the cost and risk associated with implant placement makes this unreasonable in most cases.[20]

REFERENCES

1. Torabinejad M, Anderson P, Bader J, et al. Outcomes of root canal treatment and restoration, implant-supported single crowns, fixed partial dentures, and extraction without replacement: a systematic review. J Prosthet Dent. 2007; 98: 285–311.
2. Kvist T, Reit C. Results of endodontic retreatment: a randomized clinical study comparing surgical and nonsurgical procedures. J Endod. 1999; 25: 814–7.
3. Rahbaran S, Gilthorpe MS, Harrison SD, Gulabivala K. Comparison of clinical outcome of periapical surgery in endodontic and oral surgery units of a teaching dental hospital: a retrospective study. Oral Surg Oral Med Oral Pathol Oral Radiol Endod. 2001; 91: 700–9.
4. Ng YL, Mann V, Rahbaran S, Lewsey J, Gulabivala K. Outcome of primary root canal treatment: systematic review of the literature – Part 2. Influence of clinical factors. Int Endod J. 2008; 41: 6–31.
5. Nair PNR. On the causes of persistent apical periodontitis: a review. Int Endod J. 2006; 39: 249–81.
6. Tronstad L, Barnett F, Cervone F. Periapical bacterial plaque in teeth refractory to endodontic treatment. Endod Dent Traumatol. 1990; 6: 73–7.
7. Nair PN. Cholesterol as an aetiological agent in endodontic failures–a review. Aust Endod J. 1999; 25: 19–26.
8. Nair PN, Sjogren U, Krey G, Sundqvist G. Therapy-resistant foreign body giant cell granuloma at the periapex of a root-filled human tooth. J Endod. 1990; 16: 589–95.
9. Ramachandran Nair PN, Pajarola G, Schroeder HE. Types and incidence of human periapical lesions obtained with extracted teeth. Oral Surg Oral Med Oral Pathol Oral Radiol Endod. 1996; 81: 93–102.
10. Briggs PF, Scott BJ. Evidence-based dentistry: endodontic failure–how should it be managed? Br Dent J [Internet]. 1997; 183: 159–64.
11. Danin J, Stromberg T, Forsgren H, Linder LE, Ramskold LO. Clinical management of nonhealing periradicular pathosis. Surgery versus endodontic retreatment. Oral Surg Oral Med Oral Pathol Oral Radiol Endod. 1996; 82: 213–7.

12. Evans G, Bishop K, Renton T. Update of guidelines for surgical endodontics—the position after ten years. Br Dent J. 2012; 212: 497–8.
13. Taschieri S, Del Fabbro M, Testori T, Francetti L, Weinstein R. Endodontic surgery using 2 different magnification devices: preliminary results of a randomized controlled study. J Oral Maxillofac Surg. 2006; 64: 235–42.
14. de Chevigny C, Dao TT, Basrani BR, et al. Treatment outcome in endodontics: the Toronto study–phases 3 and 4: orthograde retreatment. J Endod. 2008; 34: 131–7.
15. Testori T, Capelli M, Milani S, Weinstein RL. Success and failure in periradicular surgery: a longitudinal retrospective analysis. Oral Surg Oral Med Oral Pathol Oral Radiol Endod. 1999; 87: 493–8.
16. Fernandez-Yanez Sanchez A, Leco-Berrocal MI, Martinez-Gonzalez JM. Metaanalysis of filler materials in periapical surgery. Med Oral Patol Oral Cir Bucal. 2008; 13: E180–5.
17. El-Swiah JM, Walker RT. Reasons for apicectomies: A retrospective study. Endod Dent Traumatol. 1996; 12: 185–91.
18. Del Fabbro M, Taschieri S, Testori T, Francetti L, Weinstein RL. Surgical versus non-surgical endodontic re-treatment for periradicular lesions. Cochrane database Syst Rev. 2007; (3): CD005511.
19. Gagliani MM, Gorni FGM, Srohmenger L. Periapical resurgery versus periapical surgery: a 5-year longitudinal comparison. Int Endodont J. 2005; 38: 320–7.
20. Setzer FC, Kim S. Comparison of long-term survival of implants and endodontically treated teeth. J Dent Res. 2014; 93: 19–26.

CHAPTER 27

A 15-Year Study of Osseointegrated Implants in the Treatment of the Edentulous Jaw

Adell R, Lekholm U, Rockler B, Brånemark PI. Int J Oral Surg. 1981; 10: 387–416.

Reviewed by Baucke van Minnen

Research Objective

The purpose of the paper was to provide a review of both the treatment methods and clinical results from 15 years (1965–1980) use of osseointegrated implants supporting a removable bridge for the rehabilitation of edentulous jaws. The review of the treatment methods was a relevant part of the study, as between 1965 and 1971 changes in the clinical procedures were frequently made. From 1971, the clinical procedures were minimally changed so the clinical results of a relatively homogenous group of patients could be readily evaluated.

Study Design and Sample Sizes

The authors categorised three groups of patients as a result of the evolution of the clinical procedures in three time periods:

I. Initial period (1965–1968), when experimental knowledge was introduced to the clinical situation.
II. Development period (1968–1971), during which certain modifications of the method were introduced, due to differences between the experimental and the clinical conditions.
III. Routine period (1971–1980), when only minor technical adjustments were made.

Indications for treatment were an edentulous state for more than 1 year with insufficient retention for a denture; the patient's inability to accept a (technically adequate) denture, or functional disturbances (e.g., severe nausea and vomiting reflexes). A total of 371 edentulous patients were treated between 1965 and 1980. In these patients, 2,768 implants were placed.

The *anchorage function* was calculated for the total number of included implants and defined as the ratio between the number of stable, osseointegrated implants supporting a bridge, in relation to the total number of installed implants.

If osseointegration was not achieved, supplementary implants were placed after removal and healing of the bone. The percentage of supplementary implants and the distribution among groups II and III were calculated.

Independent of the loss of a single implant, the bridge might remain functional, as long as it is sufficiently supported by the remaining implants. This *continuous bridge stability* was used as an important outcome measure, as for the patients, bridge stability and function are of greater interest for their total rehabilitation than the fate of an individual implant.

Several samples were taken from the whole patient group to evaluate other outcome measures:

a. From the development group (II) 17 patients were recalled for a detailed evaluation of the marginal mucosa.
b. A random sample of 43 patients was evaluated for complications.
c. There was sufficient radiological data for marginal bone loss to be analysed in 326 implants. Marginal bone loss was only measured during the routine period of the project after developing a standardised method for serial radiographic examination.

Follow-up
All consecutive cases with a follow-up of 1–15 years.

Inclusion/Exclusion Criteria
Patients with a severely resorbed maxilla with a need for augmentation were excluded and evaluated in another publication. After excluding the patients with a follow-up of less than a year, 284 patients with 1,997 implants remained.

Treatment Received
A two-stage surgical procedure was performed. For both the mandible and the maxilla, six titanium implants were placed. Locations with sufficient bone were identified by explorative drilling. The different steps of drilling and implant insertion were described in detail. Healing time was 3–4 months in the lower jaw and 5–6 months in the upper jaw. After the healing period, an abutment operation was performed. The prosthetic treatment started 2 weeks after placing the abutments. Screw-retained bridges with a gold framework and acrylic occlusal and incisal covering were placed.

Results
Anchorage function was 81% in the upper jaw and 91% in the lower jaw in the routine group after 5–9 years follow-up. These percentages were 48% and 63%, respectively, in the development group. The percentage of supplementary implants was 22% (upper jaw) and 11% (lower jaw) in the development group.

Depending on the follow-up, these percentages varied from 12 to 15% and 4 to 9%, respectively, in the routine group.

The mean clinical pocket depth was 2.6 mm in Sample A. Gingivitis was found in 7.6% of patients. Mean bone loss was 1.5 mm during the healing period and the first year after abutment connection. The risk of mechanical complications was higher in the upper jaw than in the lower jaw. Five percent of the implants (69/1,997) fractured during the study.

Despite the complications and the relatively high percentages of supplementary implants, the continuous bridge stability in the routine group was 100% in the lower jaw and 89% in the upper jaw. In the development group this was 100% and 79%.

The authors conclude that an implant-supported bridge provides a reliable oral rehabilitation method for edentulous patients.

Study Limitations

The purpose of the study was to give a review of both the treatment methods and the clinical results. The clinical results have been extensively reviewed; however, the authors do not clarify what they have changed in the surgical procedure over the years between the three study groups in this article. They demonstrate that the loss of implants and anchorage function in the development groups was higher, and that a thorough surgical procedure with minimal damage to the host tissues is important. More details are given in another publication by Brånemark et al.[1]

Length, diameter, composition, and surface characteristics of the implant, and the implant-to-abutment connection of the titanium implants are not described in detail in this study. The authors cannot be blamed for that, as in that time it was not clear that this would become important characteristics and indicators for success of implantology, especially in compromised and aesthetically challenging anatomical situations.

The title and abstract suggest that all consecutive patients in a 15-year time period were evaluated, but this was not in fact the case. Nevertheless, this is the first study with a long-term clinical follow-up of patients undergoing treatment of the edentulous jaw with osseointegrated implants.

Relevant Studies

The experimental study of osseointegration was published by Brånemark in 1969.[2] This 15-year follow-up study was published in a time when there was still debate about the concept of osseointegrated implants. The proof of osseointegration was not the objective of this publication; nevertheless, the authors used many arguments to convince the reader of the presence of osseointegration. The publication can be seen as a plea for osseointegration in a time period where other scientists were still evaluating other implantology concepts (e.g., with implants developing a pseudo-periodontium after insertion).

In general, collecting long-term follow-up data of implantology studies is challenging. Treatment concepts are changing rapidly, and therefore it can be difficult to define a homogenous patient group for long-term follow-up.

This is the first study with a long-term clinical follow-up of consecutive patients undergoing treatment of the edentulous jaw with osseointegrated implants. The authors concluded that the treatment can be performed with a reliable prognosis. Although their study has limitations, mainly because of the changing treatment strategies during the study period, the past decades have shown that the authors were indeed correct in their conclusions.

The "anchorage function" can be described as survival of functional implants and resembles the "implant survival," which is nowadays often calculated in comparable clinical publications. Implant survival in a noncompromised patient currently approaches 100% after 1 year. This publication described an improvement of anchorage function from 48% to 81% in the upper jaw and from 63% to 91% in the lower jaw, which is an admirable improvement.

Many aspects of the treatment protocol described in this publication are currently still being used. First, the concept of screw-shaped titanium implants is still vital. Since 1981, many changes in the titanium screw-shaped implants have been proposed with regard to diameter, length, thread, abutment and prosthetic connections, type of alloy, and surface characteristics. They all have been extensively reviewed in clinical practice and have led to a further improvement of implant survival and aesthetics and a decline in mechanical complications.

The indications for implant treatment of the edentulous patients have hardly changed over the years. The treatment strategies have, however, undergone major developments. Varying prosthetic solutions with overdentures and fixed and removable bridges have been performed on a varying number of implants. In general, the number of implants used to support the prosthesis has gradually declined over the years as a result of reliable osseointegration and mechanical improvement of the implants themselves.

Most of the steps in the surgical procedure are still in some way a part of the current surgical procedures. It remains of vital importance not to harm the recipient bone by cooling and stepwise drilling. Surgeons still look for the locations with sufficient amount of bone, only not by explorative drilling but by 3D radiology and virtual planning. Alignment of the implants is still important, but modern guided surgery has replaced the direction indicators in many clinical situations. Obvious differences in the clinical procedures exist as well. Nowadays, many implants are placed in a one-stage procedure, while the authors followed a strict two-stage procedure. Early or direct restoration and loading have become possible in selected cases, whereas the authors stress the importance of a long healing time.

Whilst many aspects of dental implantology have evolved in the last half century,[3] the publications by the Brånemark group remain the source of these developments.

REFERENCES

1. Brånemark PI, Hansson BO, Adell R, et al. Osseointegrated implants in the treatment of the edentulous jaw. Experience from a 10-year period. Scand J Plast Reconstr Surg Suppl. 1977; 16: 1–132.
2. Brånemark PI, Adell R, Breine U, et al. Intra-osseous anchorage of dental prostheses. I. Experimental studies. Scand J Plast Reconstr Surg. 1969; 3: 81–100.
3. Lindhe J, Lang NP (Eds.). Clinical Periodontology and Implant Dentistry. Oxford: Blackwell Publishing Ltd., 2015.

CHAPTER 28

Osteonecrosis of the Jaws Associated with the Use of Bisphosphonates: A Review of 63 Cases

Ruggiero SL, Mehrotra B, Rosenberg TJ, Engroff SL. J Oral Maxillofac Surg. 2004; 62: 527–34.

Reviewed by Simon Rogers and Derek Lowe

Research Question/Objective

At the Oral and Maxillofacial Surgery Departments of the Long Island Jewish Medical Center in New York and of the University of Maryland, Baltimore, a growing number of patients between 2001 and 2003 were being referred for evaluation and management of "refractory osteomyelitis" of varying duration. The typical presentation was a non-healing extraction socket or exposed jawbone with progression to sequestrum formation associated with localised swelling and purulent discharge. Up to this point, this rare clinical scenario was seen only in patients who had received radiation therapy and who accounted for one or two cases per year. The purpose of the study was to perform a retrospective chart review of these patients.

Study Design

A retrospective case series chart review of all patients presenting between February 2001 and November 2003 with the diagnosis of osteonecrosis or osteomyelitis of the jaw.

Sample Size

A total of 63 patients were identified with such a diagnosis.

Follow-up

Not applicable.

Inclusion/Exclusion

Patients who presented with a diagnosis of osteonecrosis or osteomyelitis of the jaw were included in the review. Patients who had a prior history of radiation therapy to the jaw region or neoplastic disease that directly involved the jaws were excluded from the review.

Intervention or Treatment Received

Most patients had surgical procedures to remove all of the involved bone.

Results

All 63 patients, 45 females, and 18 males, mean age (range): 63 (43–89) years had received intravenous bisphosphonates for at least a year and 7 were on chronic oral bisphosphonate therapy. All were actively receiving either pamidronate or zoledronic acid at monthly intervals, with 14 patients having started with pamidronate but subsequently switching to zoledronic acid. The duration of the bisphosphonate therapy at presentation ranged from 6 to 48 months.

Oncological diagnoses at presentation comprised multiple myeloma (28 patients), breast cancer (21 patients), prostate cancer (3 patients), lung cancer (1 patient), uterine leiomyosarcoma (1 patient), plasmacytoma (1 patient), and leukaemia (1 patient). Seven patients were diagnosed with osteoporosis without any history of malignant disease or chemotherapy exposure. Twenty-four patients (38%) presented with maxillary bone involvement (20 unilateral and 4 bilateral) and 40 (63%) had mandibular bone involvement (37 unilateral and 3 bilateral). One patient presented with exposed and necrotic bone in all four quadrants. All patients had radiographic or nuclear scan evidence of metastatic osteolytic bone lesions.

Typical presenting lesions were either a non-healing extraction socket or exposed jawbone; both were refractory to conservative debridement and antibiotic therapy. All involved sites had previously undergone biopsy to rule out metastatic disease. No patients had received radiation therapy to the region surrounding the jawbones. Typical presenting symptoms were pain and exposed bone at the site of a previous tooth extraction. However, 9/63 patients (14%) with no history of a recent dentoalveolar procedure presented with spontaneous exposure and necrosis of the alveolar bone. Radiographs routinely showed regions of mottled bone, consistent with sequestrum formation. Chronic maxillary sinusitis secondary to necrotic bone and an oroantral fistula were evident in several patients with posterior maxillary involvement. On microscopic examination, all of the specimens consisted of necrotic bone with associated bacterial debris and granulation tissue. Culture results consistently revealed normal oral flora. Six patients had radiographic signs of osteolysis before the extraction of teeth, which suggested involvement of the alveolar bone before extraction.

Most patients required surgical procedures to remove all of the involved bone, and 75% had a sequestrectomy; other procedures involved marginal mandibular resection, segmental mandibular resection, and partial or complete maxillectomy. Two patients received hyperbaric oxygen therapy (30 one-hour sessions) before undergoing a marginal mandibular resection of necrotic bone, and despite having vascularised bone at the resection margins, there was progressive necrosis most likely requiring a segmental resection. Two asymptomatic patients with regions of exposed and necrotic bone were followed and treated conservatively with local wound care and irrigations. One patient with metastatic uterine leiomyosarcoma presented with a large sequestered segment of the right maxilla that had spontaneously exfoliated, resulting in a large oroantral communication. Stopping bisphosphonate treatment did not have a major impact on the progression of this process. Five patients had persistent bone necrosis and even developed new regions of exposed bone despite being removed from bisphosphonate therapy by their oncologists.

Study Limitations

The method was a case note review of patients presenting to two hospitals during "the past 3 years." Case selection will be liable to referral bias and case identification and data details limited by the retrospective nature of the study. The assumption is that this was a consecutive case series, but this is not explicitly stated.

It is clear from the summary in the paper that the majority of bisphosphonates were administered intravenously (numerator), but there are no numbers on how many were treated (denominator) for the purpose of quantifying risk. Having so many cases related to intravenous administration would suggest an increased relative risk over oral bisphosphonates. There are some minor inconsistencies in the number of patients noted within the paper, between text and tables, for example, cancer type, site, treatments, and use of hyperbaric oxygen. There is a lack of detail in variables such as length of follow-up following surgery, use of antibiotics, chlorhexidine mouthwash, impact of treatment on patient symptoms, and function. However, the paper was enhanced by the inclusion of a clinical photograph, radiographs, and a photomicrograph of a sequestrum. As a case series, it lacks meaningful follow-up data in respect to analysis of outcome by any variations in intervention.

Relevant Studies

The year 2003 saw several case histories and preliminary communication issued by the Division of Oral and Maxillofacial Surgery at the University of Miami School of Medicine to highlight the emergence of a new form of "osteomyelitis," specifically avascular necrosis of the jaw related to bisphosphonates.[1,2] However, it was the series of 63 cases by Ruggiero and colleagues published in 2004 that really was the first substantial paper that brought home to the clinical fraternity the theretofore unrecognised and underreported serious adverse effect of bisphosphonates. At the time of publication, there were still a considerable number of clinicians who had never seen a case and questioned it as a clinical entity.

Since the publication of this paper, there has been a better understanding of incidence, national rates, clinical characteristics, risk factors, and coexisting conditions.[3] An international multicentre study from 22 secondary care centres in seven countries emphasised the need to develop risk-reduction strategies aimed at either assessing or modulating the risk of osteonecrosis of the jaws (ONJ) associated with bisphosphonates.[4]

Another area to consider in the often-used bisphosphonate-related osteonecrosis of the jaws (BRONJ) terminology is that this has now been changed to antiresorptive drug-related osteonecrosis of the jaws (ARONJ) and medication-related osteonecrosis of the jaw (MRONJ).[5,6] This reflects the association of necrosis with the emergence of newer drugs such as denosumab that have a different mode of action and pharmacotherapeutics profile.

Studies exploring genetic predisposition have also helped understanding its pathogenesis findings that inflammation and infection might play an important role.[7]

There is no doubt about the benefits to patients of antiresorptive treatment, but in spite of the passage of time since Ruggiero first published the 63 cases and a substantial number of papers on this issue, there are still a lot of unanswered questions related to risk versus benefit of ARONJ and the most effective treatment.[8,9]

REFERENCES

1. Wang J, Goodger NM, Pogrel MA. Osteonecrosis of the jaws associated with cancer chemotherapy. J Oral Maxillofac Surg. 2003; 61: 1104–7.
2. Marx RE. Pamidronate (Aredia) and zoledronate (Zometa) induced avascular necrosis of the jaws: a growing epidemic. J Oral Maxillofac Surg. 2003; 61: 1115–7.
3. Rogers SN, Palmer NO, Lowe D, Randall C. United Kingdom nationwide study of avascular necrosis of the jaws including bisphosphonate-related necrosis. Br J Oral Maxillofac Surg. 2015; 53: 176–82.
4. Fung P, Bedogni G, Bedogni A, et al. Time to onset of bisphosphonate-related osteonecrosis of the jaws: a multicentre retrospective cohort study. Oral Dis. 2017; 23: 477–83.
5. Moore A, Renton T, Taylor T, et al. Oral surgery: ARONJ masterclass. Br Dent J. 2014; 216: 488–9.
6. Aljohani S, Fliefel R, Ihbe J, et al. What is the effect of anti-resorptive drugs (ARDs) on the development of medication-related osteonecrosis of the jaw (MRONJ) in osteoporosis patients: a systematic review. J Craniomaxillofac Surg. 2017; 45: 1493–1502.
7. Stockmann P, Nkenke E, Englbrecht M, et al. Major histocompatibility complex class II polymorphisms are associated with the development of anti-resorptive agent-induced osteonecrosis of the jaw. J Craniomaxillofac Surg. 2013; 41: 71–5.

8. Patel V, McLeod N, Rogers SN, Brennan PA. Bisphosphonate osteonecrosis of the jaw—a literature review of UK policies versus international policies on bisphosphonates, risk factors and prevention. Br J Oral Maxillofac Surg. 2011; 49: 251–7.
9. McLeod N, Patel V, Kusanale A, Rogers SN, Brennan PA. Bisphosphonate osteonecrosis of the jaw – a literature review of UK policies versus international policies on the management of bisphosphonate osteonecrosis of the jaws. Br J Oral Maxillofac Surg. 2011; 49: 335–42.

CHAPTER 29

The Anatomical Location of the Mandibular Canal: Its Relationship to the Sagittal Ramus Osteotomy

Rachel J, Ellis E 3rd, Fonseca RJ. Int J Adult Orthodon Orthognath Surg. 1986; 1: 37–47.

Reviewed by Stephen Walsh

Research Question/Objective

To define the anatomical position of the mandibular canal and thereby its neurovascular bundle and to relate the findings to the sagittal split osteotomy procedure. There were no previous studies that had provided information about the mediolateral position of the neurovascular bundle.

Study Design

Forty-five dried adult Asian (sex and age unknown) intact mandibles with nearly complete dentitions were sectioned—first along the midline (to create a hemimandible) and then at defined standardised points perpendicular to the sagittal plane: just posterior to mental foramen, just anterior to mandibular foramen and at three equal intervals between these two sites. The size and position of the mandibular canal in relation to the lingual cortex, buccal cortex and the inferior border of the mandible was measured with calipers.

Sample Size

Forty-five mandibles—Analysis of the 90 resulting hemimandibles showed no statistical difference in results between left and right sides and allowed therefore 90 specimens to be used for calculation as a single group.

Results

The authors demonstrated that the mandibular canal is in its most lingual position at the lingula and most buccal position just prior to exiting the mental foramen. The distance from the lateral canal wall to the medial aspect of the buccal cortex was significantly different in each section, with the first molar region being the thickest (4.05 mm +/–1.10 mm) and then followed by the second molar region, with a significant reduction in distance in the other areas. The findings demonstrated that the mandible in the first and second molar regions offers the most medullary bone between canal and cortical plate.

In combination with the results demonstrating that the buccal cortical plate was also thickest at the furcation or distal half of the first, and second molar, these areas are the safest to both make and instrument vertical cuts when performing a sagittal split osteotomy. This helps to avoid direct injury to the nerve during instrumentation (and perhaps avoid a buccal plate fracture with bone thickness sufficient to support instrumentation).

It is worth remembering that historically the sagittal split "vertical" or "buccal" cut had evolved with time from a much more posteriorly directed cut (to the angle or behind it) to slowly make its way forward along the body of the ramus.[2,3] This research has demonstrated the safety and logic behind this evolution.

The study also supports the avoidance of the third molar area (advocated by some authors at the time for performing the vertical cut[3]), as there is less room for error here because the nerve lies closer to the buccal cortical plate.

The authors use the study to support extending the buccal plate osteotomy cut to the area between the first and second molars because they demonstrated that:

1. The buccal cortical plate is thickest here.
2. The total mandibular body width is thickest here.
3. The distance between the inner aspect of the buccal plate and the mandibular canal is consistently greatest at this location.

The study also demonstrated that the most inferior point of the canal is at the distal half of the first molar tooth and NOT at the mental foramen. This is of particular relevance when you are performing a genioplasty. The operator must ensure that the genioplasty osteotomy lies well below the mental foramen to ensure the nerve is not sectioned inferior to and proximal to the mental foramen when you are performing the horizontal cut.

Study Limitations

This paper is from 1986, and the techniques and instrumentation available at the time may not match those currently in clinical use; for example, power saws and drills are perhaps more efficient in size, manoeuvreability, and cutting ability and the advent of piezoelectric instruments may negate much of the potential direct trauma to the nerve in this area of practice in due course.[1] The basis of the splitting technique, although modified by individual practitioners, is however still broadly the same.

The authors discuss critical papers and modifications of osteotomy techniques largely from the 1960s and 1970s aimed at trying to reduce complications as this procedure was gaining acceptance and increasingly used in the world of orthognathic treatment. The surgeon of the 21st century will therefore need to place this article in context, as many of the procedural modifications discussed are no longer in clinical practice.

The mandibles were all from Asian patients, so this research may not translate to other races. The sex and age of the patients were unknown, as were the jaw/occlusal relationships, and may not therefore represent cases from which a sagittal split osteotomy is likely to be undertaken in real clinical scenarios.

Relevant Studies

Mandibular osteotomies are undertaken in many different forms, but the most frequently used procedure is based on the sagittal split osteotomy, initially described by Obwegeser and Trauner in 1955.[2,3]

Several important modifications have been described including by DalPont,[4] who described the vertical cut through the lateral cortex and the shortened horizontal cut to the lingula, also discussed by Hunsuck.[5]

Inferior alveolar nerve injury occurs in 31–37% of patients following a sagittal split osteotomy and may be associated with medial retraction of the soft tissues medial to the ramus, the buccal cortical cut, the splitting of the bone, or fixation.[6–9] Yoshida et al. and Yamamoto et al. found that neurosensory disturbance was associated with the proximity of the nerve to the lateral cortex.[10,11] For this reason, understanding of the position of the nerve when making the surgical cuts and splitting the mandible is important. Modifications in instrumentation and technique have been proposed to reduce the incidence of inferior alveolar nerve injury, but to date there is no robust evidence supporting one technique over another.[12]

It was thought that the use of piezoelectric surgery would reduce the incidence of neurosensory deficit with mandibular osteotomies, but the evidence for this is currently lacking.[13]

REFERENCES

1. Pagotto LEC, de Santana Santos T, de Vasconcellos SJA, Santos JS, Martins-Filho PRS. Piezoelectric versus conventional techniques for orthognathic surgery: systematic. J Craniomaxillofac Surg. 2017; 45: 1607–13.
2. Obwegeser H, Trauner R. Zur operationtechnick bei der progenie und anderen unterkieferanomalien. Dtsch Zahn Mund Kieferheilkd. 1955; 23: H1–H2.
3. Obwegeser HL. Orthognathic surgery and a tale of how three procedures came to be: a letter to the next generations of surgeons. Clin Plast Surg. 2007; 34: 331–55.
4. DalPont G. Retromolar osteotomy for the correction of prognathism. J Oral Surg Anesth Hosp Dent Serv. 1961; 19: 42–7.

5. Hunsuck EE. Modified intraoral sagittal splitting technique for the correction of mandibular prognathism. J Oral Surg. 1968; 26: 249–52.

6. McLeod NMH, Bowe DC. Nerve injury associated with orthognathic surgery; Part 2: inferior alveolar nerve. Br J Oral Maxillofac Surg. 2016; 54: 366–71.

7. White RP, Peters PB, Costich ER, Page HL Jr. Evaluation of sagittal split-ramus osteotomy in 17 patients. J Oral Surg. 1969; 27: 851–5.

8. Guernsey LH, DeChamplain RW. Sequelae and complications of the intraoral sagittal osteotomy in the mandibular rami. Oral Surg. 1971; 32: 176–92.

9. Lemke RR, Rugh JD, Van Sickels J, Bays RA, Clark GM. Neurosensory differences after wire and rigid fixation in patients with mandibular advancement. J Oral Maxillofac Surg. 2000; 58: 1354–9.

10. Yoshida T, Nagamine T, Kobayashi T, et al. Impairment of the inferior alveolar nerve after sagittal split osteotomy. J Craniomaxillofac Surg. 1989; 17: 271–7.

11. Yamamoto R, Nakamura A, Ohno K, Michi KI. Relationship of the mandibular canal to the lateral cortex of the mandibular ramus as a factor in the development of neurosensory disturbance after bilateral sagittal split osteotomy. J Oral Maxillofac Surg. 2002; 60: 490–5.

12. Brusati R, Fiamminghi L, Sesenna E, Gazzotti A. Functional disturbance of the inferior alveolar nerve after sagittal osteotomy of the mandibular ramus: operating technique for prevention. J Maxillofac Surg. 1981; 9: 123–5.

13. Rude K, Svensson P, Starch-Jensen T. Neurosensory disturbances after bilateral sagittal split osteotomy using piezoelectric surgery: a systematic review. J Oral Maxillofac Surg. 2019; 77: 380–90.

CHAPTER 30

A Modification of the Pterygoid Plate Separation in Low-Level Maxillary Osteotomies

Trimble LD, Tideman H, Stoelinga PJW. J Oral Maxillofac Surg. 1983; 41: 544–6.

Reviewed by Jan de Lange

Research Question/Objective

Description of a modified technique to separate the pterygoid plate in a Le Fort 1 osteotomy.

Study Design

Descriptive.

Intervention or Treatment Received

The article is a technical note describing a modified technique that can be applied during a Le Fort I procedure. The initial access incision and bone cuts are fairly standard for a low-level Le Fort I osteotomy. If the maxillary third molar is not present, or impacted very high, a chisel is applied to the alveolus 0.5 cm behind the second molar and angled at a slightly posterior, medial, and superior direction. A finger is placed on the palatal aspect of the tuberosity and the chisel struck until it can be felt against the palatal finger. If the third molar is present and impacted, a vertical incision is made distal to the second molar and the tooth extracted through this, with the chisel then applied in a similar manner. The maxilla is then down-fractured in a standard manner.

Study Limitations

This is a technical note introducing a modified technique for Le Fort 1 osteotomies. As such, it contains the description of the technique without any clinical research associated with the technique.

Relevant Studies

Trimble, Tideman, and Stoelinga were not the first to suggest a pterygoid plate separation through the maxillary tuberosity. This was already described by Dupont et al.[1] In this earlier description, a chisel was inserted through the cheek to reach the maxillary tuberosity, while Trimble described positioning the chisel through the oral cavity without the use of a separate access incision. According to the authors, the main advantages of the new technique were the much lower chance of pterygoid plate fracture and a decreased risk of bleeding of the maxillary artery. However, they did not present any clinical research to support this hypothesis, and it was not until 2015 that a small randomised clinical trial (RCT) was published to support some of their earlier claims.

Dadwal et al.[2] performed a study in which they randomised between the classical separation between the maxilla/pterygoid plate and the technique as described by Trimble et al. In the group using the Trimble technique, post-operative CT showed no pterygoid plate fractures, whereas fractures were found in 3 out of 8 sides using the classical pterygoid separation technique. Fractures occurred in patients in whom the thickness of the pterygomaxillary junction was less than or equal to 3.6 mm. There were no massive bleeds or other complications such as skull base fractures in either group. The Trimble technique therefore can be regarded as a safer method, especially regarding unwanted fractures in the pterygoid plates. Unfortunately, this RCT only included eight patients and therefore the conclusions have to be interpreted with some care.

Other research on this topic has mainly focused on fractures of the pterygoid plates and the use of different tools to avoid them. Stajcic showed that a more curved chisel would help to decrease the number of pterygoid plate fractures, while Lanigan and Guest advised to not use any chisel at all but instead utilise a micro-oscillating saw.[3,4] Both these studies were done on cadavers and only Lanigan and Guest included the technique described by Trimble. They found that the conventional technique resulted in ideal separations in only 3/20 sides (15%), low-level fractures in 12/20 sides (60%), and high-level fractures in 5/20 sides (25%). The Trimble technique resulted in ideal separations in 9/20 sides (45%), low-level fractures in 6/20 sides (30%), and high-level fractures in 5/20 sides (25%). While the Trimble technique led to an improvement in the incidence of ideal separations, it still included a high incidence of high-level pterygoid plate fractures.

At the beginning of the 1990s, a group from Canada published two papers on the separation of the maxilla and pterygoid plate using no chisel or osteotome at all. In their first article a group of 500 patients was presented in which this technique was used.[5] There were no fractures of the pterygoid plates, and they experienced no other major complications. In their second article, a comparison between using an osteotome in the classic way and not using any osteotome was made.[6] The conclusion based on the results of the study was that there is no more risk in performing Le Fort I osteotomy without a chisel than with using one to accomplish pterygomaxillary separation. It was also found that avoiding the use of chisel will not prevent pterygoid plate fracture. Unfortunately, the method as described by Trimble et al. was not included in this study, and therefore it remains a question whether or not the Trimble technique would result in a different complication rate compared to not using any chisel at all.

Complications associated with Le Fort I osteotomy, such as haemorrhage from the sphenopalatine, descending palatine and maxillary arteries, arteriovenous fistulae, skull base fracture, cranial nerve injury, blindness, ophthalmic complications, and internal carotid artery injury, have all been reported in the literature. Often, these complications have been attributed to the nonideal separation of the pterygomaxillary junction. It has been suggested that unfavourable separation between the pterygoid plates and the posterior maxillary walls may result in horizontal or oblique fractures of the pterygoid plates, and that this is a major contributing factor to these complications. Fortunately, pterygoid plate fractures mostly occur independent of any other complications. These independent pterygoid plate fractures are rarely a problem, although the fractured segments can interfere with the mobilisation of the maxilla during advancement or setback. The technique that was described by Trimble as a modification of the earlier publication by Dupont is a method that reduces the number of pterygoid plate fractures and therefore the possibility of more severe complications during a Le Fort I osteotomy.

In conclusion, the Trimble technique is a modification of the method that was published in 1974 by Dupont. It has proved to be a valuable variation of the standard Le Fort I procedure and should be applied in order to reduce the risk of pterygoid plate fractures and more severe complications associated with these fractures.

REFERENCES

1. Dupont C, Ciaburro H, Prévost Y. Simplifying the le fort I type of maxillary osteotomy. Plas Recon Surg. 1974; 54: 142–7.
2. Dadwal H, Shanmugasundaram S, Krishnakumar Raja VB. Preoperative and postoperative CT scan assessment of pterygomaxillary junction in patients undergoing Le Fort I Osteotomy: comparison of pterygomaxillary dysjunction technique and Trimble technique – a pilot study. Maxillofac Oral Surg. 2015; 14: 713–9.
3. Stajcic Z. Altering the angulation of a curved osteotome-does it have effects on the type of pterygomaxillary disjunction in Le Fort I osteotomy? Int J Oral Maxillofac Surg. 1991; 20: 301–3.
4. Lanigan DT, Guest P. Alternative approaches to pterygomaxillary separation. Int J Oral Maxillofac Surg. 1993; 22: 131–8.
5. Precious DS, Morrison A, Ricard D. Pterygomaxillary separation without the use of an osteotome. J Oral Maxillofac Surg. 1991; 49: 95–9.
6. Precious DS, Goodday RH, Bourget L, Skulsky FG. Pterygoid plate fracture in Le Fort I osteotomy with and without pterygoid chisel: a computed tomography scan evaluation of 58 patients. J Oral Maxillofac Surg. 1993; 51: 151–3.

CHAPTER 31

Posterior Maxillary Surgery: Its Place in the Treatment of Dentofacial Deformities

West RA, Epker BN. J Oral Surg. 1972; 30: 562–3.

Reviewed by Greg J Knepil and Graham R Oliver

Research Question/Objective

The paper explores the role of posterior maxillary segmental osteotomy in the management of dentofacial deformity. The authors reviewed contemporaneous techniques and outcomes of segmenting and repositioning of the posterior segment of the maxilla, without the use of a Le Fort I down fracture. It describes indications and gives a detailed description of several novel surgical techniques, with results and complications arising from their own experience, and those described by Schuchardt, Kufner, and Perko.[1-3]

Study Design

The results are derived from a nonrandomised case series of patients undergoing surgery between 1968 and 1972.

Number of Patients Included in the Study

Twelve patients were included in the case series, although only three are described in detail.

Follow-up

Less than 3 years.

Inclusion/Exclusion Criteria

A variety of patients with dentofacial deformity were identified using clinical and photographic evaluation, dental radiographic examination with cephalometric analysis, and dental study models.

Inclusion criteria were posterior maxillary alveolar hyperplasia, total maxillary alveolar hyperplasia, bilateral/unilateral crossbite, and distal repositioning of the posterior maxillary alveolar fragment to provide space for an impacted tooth.

Patients who met the inclusion criteria but were excluded from the case series were not described.

Ethical approval for trial of these novel surgical techniques was not described.

Intervention or Treatment Received

Four indications for posterior maxillary surgery were described:

1. Posterior maxillary hyperplasia with an open bite and satisfactory lip-to-tooth relationship and increase in lower anterior face height.
2. Total maxillary alveolar hyperplasia, with an increase in vertical dimension and maxillary protrusion.
3. Bilateral or unilateral maxillary crossbite, which may exist in isolation as the only dentofacial deformity or in combination with other deformities such as cleft.
4. Distal repositioning of the posterior maxillary alveolus to create space for an unerupted maxillary canine or premolar.

Four different techniques for surgical repositioning of the posterior maxilla were presented:

1. The Schuchardt technique[1] where a palatal flap raised from the gingival margin and horizontal buccal sulcus mucosal flaps are raised to facilitate a three-sided osteotomy with the final posterior side in the pterygoid area of bony union being fractured with blunt force applied through an occlusal wafer.
2. The Kufner technique[2] performs osteotomies entirely through a horizontal buccal incision and osteotomies are undertaken with drills and chisels. An ostectomy is performed on the lateral osteotomy to facilitate access to the medial wall of the maxillary sinus, which is then osteotomised with a bur. The pterygoid osteotomy is performed with a curved osteotome, and the osteotomised posterior segment is impacted into the maxillary sinus.
3. The Perko technique[3] modifies the Schuchardt technique and uses a vertical mucoperiosteal incision in the buccal sulcus at the premolar region, which is then tunneled posteriorly to facilitate buccal osteotomies. A separate Y-shaped palatal mucosal incision is made in the midline to raise a palatal flap to access the palatal osteotomies. Another key difference between these two techniques is the exact positioning of the medial osteotomy in the palate. where Schuchardt makes the osteotomy in the palatine bone overlying the maxillary sinus and Perko makes the osteotomy in the palatal bone adjacent to the vomer. The resultant impaction by Perko reduces the size of the nasal airway, where Schuchardt reduces the osteotomized segment into the maxillary sinus and should preserve the nasal airway.

4. The authors went on to describe their own technique, which included osteotomy and repositioning of the anterior maxillary segment. They described the use of three incisions: one horizontal incision in each buccal sulcus posteriorly from premolar to tuberosity and a single vertical incision in the midline of the labial sulcus. These incisions are connected by tunnelling in the subperiosteal plane. The posterior osteotomy is similar to that described by Kufner. After the posterior segment has been mobilised, the anterior segment is approached from the buccal sulcus, and if necessary, the anterior nasal spine is reduced to prevent buckling of the cartilaginous septum.

Results

The preoperative and postoperative results of three surgical cases were presented in detail in the discussion with photographic images, anatomical line drawings of surgical techniques, and relevant anatomical effects of surgery.

No significant complications were reported; however, reference was made to the authors' earlier work in which a canine and associated regional alveolus was lost, in their opinion most likely due to devitalisation of the area.

The authors also reference the challenge in assessing surgical stability based on the short follow-up period; however, they note greater concern of relapse in relation to the two-stage technique.

Study Limitations

This study is limited by the very small sample size, which was further reduced by the variety of the dentofacial deformities treated, making this largely an illustrative non-evidence-based discussion paper. Furthermore, no case was followed up for longer than 3 years, and as such long-term stability cannot be assessed. Much of the discussion in the paper is derived from preceding studies involving larger numbers of patients, and this paper was subsequently cited by later studies, which had larger sample sizes and more detail regarding stability and complications.

Relevant Studies

Segmental maxillary osteotomies were first reported by Günter Cohn-Stock in 1921[4]; which only included osteotomy and retraction of the anterior alveolus. The surgical techniques described in the paper show the first developed techniques for segmental posterior maxillary osteotomies.[1-3] Schuchardt's early two-stage process was criticised, though, for early union of the osteotomy site resulting in more difficult movements and less stability. This was later developed into a single-stage technique[2,5]; however, there were recurrent issues related to segment vascularisation. William H. Bell was key to further exploration of maxillary blood supply and revascularisation.[6-8]

Current Management of Each Deformity

Posterior and total maxillary alveolar hyperplasia are now most commonly treated with a Le Fort I osteotomy including a differential posterior impaction, allowing for autorotation of the mandible to close an anterior open bite. This follows on from the work of Obwegeser[9,10] and simplifies the treatment to require the orthodontist to simply level the occlusal plane pre-surgery, and allow the surgeon to keep the maxilla in a single piece. Previously to achieve this, the maxilla required sectioning into multiple fragments, thereby increasing surgical complexity and complications. However, segmental surgery still has its place; it is most often employed when there is a natural step in the maxillary arch resulting in different vertical heights of posterior and anterior segments. This segmental approach also has the benefit of allowing surgical posterior expansion for correction of transverse deficiencies. Stability can be improved with pre-surgical orthodontics to open the bite further resulting in postoperative relapse in favourable direction and consequently further closure of the bite.

In modern practice, and referenced in this article, transverse discrepancies in the presence of a significant vertical or antero-posterior discrepancy can often be corrected in the pre-surgical orthodontic phase, allowing for appropriate arch coordination at the time of surgery. In cases where there is transverse coordination issue beyond the limits of orthodontics alone, then surgical expansion is indicated.[11,12] As reported in the article, this can be carried out as a segmental procedure; however, surgically assisted rapid maxillary/palatal expansion (SARME/SARPE) has become the mainstay for surgical maxillary expansion.[13,14] This may well be due to its basis and familiarity to a subtotal Le Fort I osteotomy; however, there is no agreed ideal surgical approach with variations based on release of the mid-palatal suture, pterygoid disjunction, length of corticotomy cuts, and type of distractor.[15] The evidence appears to suggest that a more invasive approach results in more predictable expansion with fewer complications.[15] Stability of any expansion-based procedure remains a key concern reported both in the article and in modern techniques.[16]

Distal repositioning of the posterior maxillary alveolus is suggested for increasing arch length for the management of orthodontic crowding, namely premolar or canine crowding. The authors acknowledge the need for this is rare and most issues can be managed orthodontically; however, they suggest its use in older patients where distal orthodontic tooth movement is more challenging. Notwithstanding this, the need for segmental maxillary surgery is lessened by the advancement of orthodontic techniques and mechanics, resulting in ever more achievable tooth movements and importantly greater acceptability to patients. The long-standing issues with all orthodontic and surgical movements are stability.

REFERENCES

1. Schuchardt K. Experiences with the surgical treatment of deformities of the jaws: prognathia, micrognathia and open bite. In Wallace AB (Ed.): International Society of Plastic Surgeons. Second Congress. London: E & S Livingstone, 1959.
2. Kufner J. Experience with a modified procedure for correction of open bite Transactions of the Third International Conference of Oral Surgery. London, E & S Livingstone, 1970. (conference paper).
3. Hargis HW. Personal Communication, 1971.
4. Wolfe SA. Günther Cohn-Stock, M.S., D.D.S., father of maxillary orthognathic surgery. J Carnio-Maxillofacial Surg. 1989; 17: 331–4.
5. Kufner J. Nove notedy chirurgickeho leceni otereneho skus. Čslka Stomat. 1960; 60: 5.
6. Bell WH, Levy BM. Revascularization and bony healing after posterior maxillary osteotomy. J Oral Surg. 1971; 29: 313–20.
7. Bell WH, Levy BM. Revascularization and bony healing after posterior maxillary corticotomies. J Oral Surg. 1972; 30: 640–8.
8. Bell WH, Fonseca RJ, Kenneky JW, Lecy BM. Bone healing and revascularization after total maxillary osteotomy. J Oral Surg. 1975; 33: 253–60.
9. Obwegeser H. Surgery of the maxilla for the correction of prognathism. SSO Schweiz Monatsschr Zahnheilkd. 1965; 75: 365–74.
10. Obwegeser H. Surgical correction of small or retrodisplaced maxillae. The 'dish-face deformity'. Plast Reconstr Surg. 1969; 43: 351–65.
11. Silverstein K, Quin P. Surgically-assisted rapid palatal expansion for management of transverse maxillary deficiency. J Oral Maxillofac Surg. 1997; 55: 725–7.
12. Suri L, Taneja P. Surgically assisted rapid palatal expansion: a literature review. Am J Orthod Dentofac Orthop. 2008; 133: 290–302.
13. Haas A. The treatment of maxillary deficiency by opening the midpalatal suture. Angle Orthod. 1965; 35: 200–17.
14. Jacobs JD, Bell WH, Williams CE, Kennedy JW. Control of the transverse dimension with surgery and orthodontics. Am J Orthod. 1980; 77: 284–306.
15. Koudstaal MJ, Poort LJ, Van Der Wal KGH, et al. Surgically assisted rapid maxillary expansion (SARME): a review of the literature. Int J Oral Maxillofac Surg. 2005; 34: 709–714.
16. Lagravère MO, Major PW, Flores-Mir C. Dental and skeletal changes following surgically assisted rapid maxillary expansion. Int J Oral Maxillofac Surg. 2006; 35: 481–7.

CHAPTER 32

Sialendoscopy for the Management of Obstructive Salivary Gland Disease: A Systematic Review and Meta-Analysis

Strychowsky JE, Sommer DD, Gupta MK, Cohen N, Nahlieli O.
Arch Otolaryngol Head Neck Surg. 2012; 138: 541–7.

Reviewed by Soudeh Chegini and Mark McGurk

Research Question/Objective

To determine the efficacy and safety of sialendoscopy in the treatment of obstructive salivary gland disease in adults.

Study Design

A systematic review using PRISMA guidelines. Two authors independently performed a multiplatform search using intervention and disease-specific terms. Data was extracted directly from the published studies and electronic communication with study authors.

Sample Size

There were 132 potentially relevant studies identified of which 29 studies met the inclusion and exclusion criteria.

Follow-up

The outcomes extracted from the literature were stone location, size, use of supportive devices, success rates, incidence of sialadenectomy and other complications. Success was defined as being symptom-free and the absence of residual obstruction.

Inclusion/Exclusion Criteria

All randomised control trials and retrospective studies found using the search method above, fully published, peer reviewed, and reporting success rate were included. There was no date range placed on the publication search. Non-English language papers and non-adult studies were excluded.

Intervention or Treatment Received

The 29 included studies evaluated either sialendoscopy alone, combined open and endoscopic approaches, and the use of sialendoscopy for radio-iodine induced sialadenitis.

Results

Sialendoscopy Alone

There were 19 studies identified involving 1,213 patients. The use of supportive devices varied from balloon dilatation, grasping instruments (basket or forceps), or fragmentation (laser of lithotripsy). Heterogeneity analysis measured a Cochrane Q of 48.7 (df = 19) ($p < 0.002$) and an I^2 (inconsistence) of 61% (95% CI, 29.4–74.9%). The weighted pooled success rate was 0.86 (95% CI, 0.83–0.89). The incidence of sialadenectomy was found to be 0–11% with a trend towards reduced gland removal in more recent publications. Complications reported included mild sialadenitis, ductal wall perforation, temporary lingual nerve paresthesia, postoperative infection, and traumatic ranula.

Sialendoscopy with Combined Surgical Approach

11 studies were identified involving 374 patients. Surgical approaches ranged from small transmucosal incisions to larger transoral incisions to preauricular parotidectomy-type incisions. Heterogeneity analysis measured a Cochrane Q of 13.8 (df = 9) ($p < 0.18$) and an I^2 (inconsistence) of 27.7% (95% CI, 0–63.8%). The weighted pooled proportion of success rates was 0.93 (95% CI, 0.89–0.96). Sialadenectomy was necessary in 0–11% cases. Complications included temporary lingual nerve paresthesia, minor glandular swelling, postoperative infection, and ductal stenosis. One retrospective series of sialoliths measuring greater than 15 mm diameter reported a single case of iatrogenic partial transection of the lingual nerve.

Sialendoscopy for Radioiodine-Induced Sialadenitis

Three studies were identified involving 33 patients. Success rates ranged from 50% to 100%. No sialadenectomy or major complications were reported.

Study Limitations

The main weakness of this paper is the heterogeneity that can be inherent in systematic reviews. This includes patient demographic, site and size of stone, and cause of obstruction.

This study does not consider the learning curve required for such a procedure. Luers et al. examined this notion and reported a statistically significant improvement on mean operating time and performance rating after the first 10 and then after the first 30 patients.[1]

Relevant Studies

Katz first described the use of a mini-flexible endoscope to remove a salivary calculus with a Dormia basket.[2]

Su et al. examined functional gland recovery after sialadenoscopy in 17 patients. They illustrated statistically significant improvement in function by sialometric and scintigraphic assessment as well as the absence of difference when compared with the contralateral gland.[3] This work supports the safety of sialendoscopy on salivary gland function.

Nahlieli et al. published a 13-year sialendoscopy experience with an overall success rate of 86% for parotid, 89% submandibular sialithotomy, and 81% for stricture treatment.[4] These results are similar to the overall success rate of 86% reported in this systematic review.

Iro et al. published a multicentred prospective observational study of extracorporeal shockwave lithotripsy alone or in combination with sialendoscopy (chapter 33). Their reported success rate in the 4,691 patients was 97% and the incidence of sialadenectomy was 2.9%.[5] These are cases where sialendoscopy was used as an adjunct for stone removal.

Zenk et al. published their outcomes in treating a total of 1,154 patients with sialolithiasis. Submandibular gland stones required removal by transoral incision (92%), or sialendoscopy alone (5%) with long-term success rates ≥90%. Parotid stones were removed by sialendoscopy alone (22%), combined sialendoscopy and incision (26%), or extracorporeal shockwave lithotripsy (52%), with long-term success rates of 98%, 89%, and 79%, respectively. Four percent of cases required surgical gland excision.[6] Again, the majority of cases required the use of sialendoscopy as an adjunct rather than primary therapeutic modality.

Management algorithms for the treatment of sialoliths based on stone diameter have been previously published. Marchal and Dulguerov recommend submandibular stones smaller than 4 mm and parotid stones smaller than 3 mm are amenable to endoscopic basket or forceps retrieval. Larger stones require fragmentation.[7] The majority of sialolithiasis presenting to clinicians are stones of much larger diameter.

Witt et al. published a consensus review on the use of sialendoscopy in collaboration with the other leading authors on this technique. The proposed algorithm outlined gland sparing management of sialolithiasis. Sialendoscopy is the suggested first-line approach for the management of submandibular gland stones of less than 5 mm. This is more likely to be successful in proximally placed stones. In the management of parotid gland stones, sialendoscopy is the first-line approach for all stones less than 5 mm and proximal stones of up to 1 cm.

Sialendoscopy can then be used in conjunction with extracorporeal lithotripsy or an open surgical approach as second- and third-line options.[8]

Sialendoscopy allows direct visualisation of the salivary gland ducts and diagnosis of stones and strictures. It also allows accurate application of therapy such as gland washout, lithotripsy, or stone removal. It is in the adjunctive use that sialendoscopy can contribute to the treatment of salivary gland conditions. As shown in this systematic review and supported by other papers discussed, sialendoscopy has limited use as primary therapeutic intervention. However, the success rate is much improved when sialendoscopy is combined with other treatments; therefore, it is a valuable technique in the armamentarium of a salivary gland surgeon.

REFERENCES

1. Luers JC, Damm M, Klussmann JP, Beutner D. The learning curve of sialendoscopy with modular sialendoscopes: a single Surgeon's experience. Arch Otolaryngol Head Neck Surg. 2010; 136: 762–5.
2. Katz P. Endoscopy of the salivary glands. Ann Radiol (Paris). 1991; 34: 110–3.
3. Su YX, Xu JH, Liao GQ, et al. Salivary gland functional recovery after sialendoscopy. Laryngoscope. 2009; 119: 646–52.
4. Nahlieli O, Nakar LH, Nazarian Y, Turner MD. Sialoendoscopy: a new approach to salivary gland obstructive pathology. J Am Dent Assoc. 2006; 137: 1394–1400.
5. Iro H, Escudier MP, Nahlieli O, et al. Outcome of minimally invasive management of salivary calculi in 4,691 patients. Laryngoscope. 2009; 119: 263–8.
6. Zenk J., Koch M, Klintworth N, et al. Sialendoscopy in the diagnosis and treatment of sialolithiasis: a study on more than 1000 patients. Otolaryngol Head Neck Surg. 2012; 147: 858–63.
7. Marchal F, Dulguerov P. Sialolithiasis management: the state of the art. Arch Otolaryngol Head Neck Surg. 2003; 129: 951–6.
8. Witt RL, Iro H, Koch M, et al. Minimally invasive options for salivary calculi. Laryngoscope. 2012; 122: 1306–11.

Outcome of Minimally Invasive Management of Salivary Calculi in 4,691 Patients

*Iro H, Zenk J, Escudier M, et al. Laryngoscope. 2009;
119: 263–8.*

Reviewed by Katherine S George and Rafal Niziol

Research Question/Objective

To evaluate the application and outcome of minimally invasive techniques in the management of salivary stones based on data from five independent European centres. Minimally invasive techniques investigated were extracorporeal shock wave lithotripsy (ESWL), retrieval by basket or micro-forceps and gland-preserving surgery.

Study Design

Prospective longitudinal study of patients treated for salivary stone disease at five centres using minimally invasive techniques. Centres involved in the study were Ashkelon, Erlangen, London, Milan, and Paris. The study period was from 1990 to 2004 inclusive. Data from all centres was pooled for analysis. There were no significant differences in the demographics of the study populations between centres. Outcomes were classified as cure (stone and symptom free), partial success (symptom free with residual stone fragments), or failure.

Sample Size

In the study, 5,258 patients with 5,993 salivary stones were treated in the five centres during the study period. After application of the exclusion criteria below, data from 4,691 was analysed. These included 3,526 cases involving the submandibular gland and 1,165 the parotid gland.

Follow-up

The authors state a median follow-up of 5 years for all patients. Those who underwent ESWL and minimally invasive surgery were reviewed radiologically by ultrasound, sialography, or both, at 3–6 months.

Inclusion/Exclusion Criteria

All patients with symptomatic disease, or at least one episode of purulent sialoadenitis, with no recovery after 3 months of conservative therapy and not amenable to simple intraoral release were included in the study.

General exclusion criteria included patients that were treated conservatively, those that refused treatment, those with complete ductal stenosis, recurrent infective episodes, multiple stones that warrant gland removal, those lost to follow-up after initial assessment, or those treated with minimally invasive procedures that do not feature in the authors' final protocol.

Further exclusion criteria were applied depending on what minimally invasive procedure the patients had. Patients were excluded from the ESWL group if they had impaired coagulation or cervical spine issues hindering positioning during treatment. They were also excluded if more than two stones were present or the stones could not be located on an ultrasound scan (USS).

Patients were excluded from the basket or micro-forceps group if the calculus was known to be fixed in the duct, located in a diverticulum, more than 50% wider than the distal duct, or there was known stenosis distally.

Patients were excluded from the gland preserving surgery group if their submandibular stone was not palpable intramurally or if the parotid stone could not be located by sialendoscopy.

Intervention or Treatment Received

All patients were treated by minimally invasive techniques, with surgical removal of the submandibular or parotid gland being a last resort. Three minimally invasive techniques were analysed:

> ESWL: This was offered at four centres. It involved a minimum of 12,000 shocks administered by a lithotripter spread over three to six sessions as an outpatient. The authors documented that patients at the Erlangen centre were admitted routinely overnight. Subsequent courses of lithotripsy were prescribed if symptoms persisted.
>
> Basket or micro-forceps retrieval: Performed under fluoroscopic, radiologic, or endoscopic guidance. The duct orifice was dilated, and the stone was engaged and withdrawn through the duct opening. This was facilitated by a papillotomy.
>
> Minimally invasive surgery: In the submandibular gland this was offered where the stones were in the hilum of the gland or in the proximal duct. Techniques included exposing the sublingual gland and following the submandibular duct to the hilum of the

gland. The duct was then either laid open along its whole length or over the stone in order to remove it. With regard to parotid duct stones, minimally invasive surgery was only offered if ESWL was unsuccessful. In this case, the stone was located using a sialendoscope and either a skin incision or preauricular flap was used to extract it.

Results

A total of 3,775 (80.5%) patients were cured, partial success was reported in 782 (16.7%), and treatment failed in 134 (2.9%) patients. Of the failed treatment group, all patients had their salivary gland removed surgically.

> ESWL: A total of 2,102 patients underwent ESWL (1,364 submandibular gland and 738 parotid gland). Treatment was successful in 1,072 (50.9%) cases, of which 40.8% were submandibular and 69.8% parotid gland. Treatment was partially successful in 544 (25.9%). Of these, 248 (33.6%) patients were cured following a second round of other minimally invasive methods. Treatment failure resulting in gland removal occurred in 110 (5.2%) of cases.
>
> Basket or micro-forceps retrieval: A total of 1,522 cases were included in this group. Cure was noted in 1,394 (91.6%), partial success in 79 (5.2%), and failure in 49 (3.2%). Seventy cases of partial or failed treatment were subsequently treated by other techniques achieving cure in 66 of these. Overall cure was achieved in 1,460 (95.9%) of cases.
>
> Minimally invasive surgery: Intra oral stone release (IOSR) from submandibular gland was performed in 1,021 patients. This was successful in 949 (95.9%) of cases, with only 18 (1.9%) requiring surgical removal of the gland. Open release of parotid stones was performed in 46 cases, with cure in 42 (91%). The remaining four cases sustained damage to parotid duct and one required removal of the gland.

Study Limitations

The main limitation of the study is the relatively short follow-up with a median of "over 5 years." This could introduce inherent bias, as patients that were initially included in the partially successful group could subsequently develop a recurrence of symptoms and require gland removal.

The authors also did not give a specific figure to quantify the loss to follow-up. These patients were incorporated into the partially successful group, which amounts to 16.6% of all cases. This could introduce a level of selection bias to the results.

Relevant Studies

In 1983, Akker and Busemann-Sokole showed that salivary glands have the potential to regain function following alleviation of outflow obstruction[1] allowing minimally invasive treatment techniques to be considered a viable alternative to gland excision in the treatment of sialolithiasis.

In the paper being considered here, the authors found that in 97.2% of cases, these techniques can avoid the need for gland excision and thus the associated risks and complications.[2]

The incidence of symptomatic sialolithiasis requiring hospital admission in the United Kingdom population has been shown to be up to 59/1,000,000 per annum. This equates to 3,850 admissions per year nationally at a cost to the NHS in 1999 of £4 million.[3] The prevalence of sialolithiasis has been estimated to be 0.45%; however, postmortem studies suggest this could be as high as 1.2%, as certain patients never presented with symptoms.[4]

Since the publication of this paper, there have been numerous technical and technological advances in minimally invasive treatment for sialolithiasis. These include advances in the design of baskets, improvement in sialendoscopes, the use of intracorporeal lithotripsy and robotics.

With regard to basket retrieval of stones, Brown et al. showed that radiologically guided basket retrieval of 86 stones in 83 patients resulted in symptomatic relief in 82% of cases.[5] In their study, fluoroscopy was used to visualise the position of the basket and its deployment. The main reason for treatment failure in these cases was fixation of the stone within the duct and in one case, malfunction of the basket requiring surgical removal. To avoid this, current baskets allow the release of the stone and multiple deployments. There has also been a shift away from fluoroscopy to sialendoscopy. This removes the need for ionising radiation, allows the operator to assess the duct (and any associated pathology), and incorporates a working channel through which a basket can be used under direct vision.

Iro et al. demonstrated that ESWL was successful in 62.8% of cases, but other studies have reported success rates as low as 26% and 39.4% of cases depending on the location of the stone.[6,7] Another technological advancement is the adaptation of intracorporeal lithotripsy techniques originally developed for renal diseases. Interventional sialendoscopy incorporating intracorporeal lithotripsy can be achieved using multiple techniques: electro-hydraulic, electrokinetic, pneumatic, and laser. Although no large studies reporting outcomes exist, success rates of 66% (electro-hydraulic) to 100% (pneumatic and laser) have been reported.[8] These techniques are not free of complications. Laser lithotripsy has a 13% complication rate, mainly due to thermal injury to the duct and surrounding tissues.[9] The general consensus appears to be that ESWL should be limited to stones that are endoscopically not accessible. The effectiveness and duration of treatment of intracorporeal lithotripsy is directly correlated to the size of the stone, its location, and operator experience. Robotically assisted surgery for stone retrieval has also been reported and may be an option in the future.[10]

Overall, Iro et al.'s paper was a paradigm shift from open excision of gland to minimally invasive techniques as a treatment for symptomatic sialolithiasis. In the United Kingdom, it resulted in the centralisation of minimally invasive salivary gland services and standardisation of treatment based on treatment algorithms,[11] thus facilitating training of clinicians to improve outcomes.

REFERENCES

1. Akker HP, Busemann-Sokole E. Submandibular gland function following transoral sialolithectomy. Oral Surg Oral Med Oral Pathol. 1983; 56: 351–6.
2. Bates D, O'Brien CJ, Tikaram K, Painter DM. Parotid and submandibular sialadenitis treated by salivary gland excision. Aust N Z J Surg. 1998; 68: 120–4.
3. Escudier MP, McGurk M. Symptomatic sialoadenitis and sialolithiasis in the English population, an estimate of the cost of hospital treatment. Br Dent J. 1999; 186: 463–6.
4. Rauch S, Gorlin RJ. Diseases of the salivary glands. In Gorlin RJ, Goldman HM (Eds.): Thoma's Oral Pathology, 6th ed., vol. 2. St. Louis, MS: Mosby, 1970.
5. Brown JE, Drage NA, Escudier MP, Wilson RF, McGurk M. Minimally invasive radiologically guided intervention for the treatment of salivary calculi. Cardiovasc Intervent Radiol. 2002; 25: 352–5.
6. Schmitz S, Zengel P, Alvir I, et al. Long-term evaluation of extracorporeal shock wave lithotripsy in the treatment of salivary stones. J Laryngol Otol. 2008; 122: 165–71.
7. McGurk M, Escudier MP, Brown JE. Modern management of salivary calculi. Br J Surg. 2005; 92: 107–12.
8. Capaccio P, Torretta S, Pignataro L, Koch M. Salivary lithotripsy in the era of sialendoscopy. Acta Otorhinolaryngol Ital. 2017; 37: 113–21.
9. Durbec M, Dinkel E, Vigier S, et al. Thulium-YAG laser sialendoscopy for parotid and submandibular sialolithiasis. Lasers Surg Med. 2012; 44: 783–6.
10. Walvekar RR1, Tyler PD, Tammareddi N, Peters G. Robotic-assisted transoral removal of a submandibular megalith. Laryngoscope. 2011; 121: 534–7.
11. Koch M, Zenk J, Iro H. Algorithms for treatment of salivary gland obstructions. Otolaryngol Clin North Am. 2009; 42: 1173–92.

CHAPTER 34

Long-Term Follow-Up of over 1,000 Patients with Salivary Gland Tumours Treated in a Single Centre

Renehan A, Gleave EN, Hancock BD, Smith P, McGurk M.
Br J Surg. 1996; 83: 1750–4.

Reviewed by Stergios Doumas and Michael WS Ho

Research Question/Objective

This study examined the clinicopathological data of 1,403 patients treated for benign and malignant salivary gland neoplasms between 1947 and 1992 in a single centre. The authors added to a previous study that was published in 1979.[1] Their objectives were to report on the epidemiology and outcomes of this relatively uncommon and heterogeneous type of head and neck tumours. They specifically addressed the survival rate according to "3 histological groups" and site of tumour.

Study Design

This was a single centre retrospective cohort study. Epidemiological and pathological data were reviewed for patients that were treated for both benign and malignant salivary gland tumours (SGTs). The primary endpoint was cancer-related mortality. Kaplan-Meier curves were plotted based on: tumour subsite, histological subgroups and tumour stage according to AJCC 4th edition. Histological examinations were reviewed in the 1970s and were reclassified based on the WHO 2nd edition (1991).

Follow-up

This is variable and at least 34 years for the pleomorphic adenomas (PSA) and 25 years for PSA that underwent malignant transformation.

Inclusion/Exclusion Criteria

Histologically confirmed tumours of epithelial origin.

Sample Size

A total of 1,403 patients with 1,432 SGTs or tumour-like lesions were assessed. In total, 1,194 tumours of epithelial origin were the subject of this study. Several other types of tumours which would have been included within the WHO classification 2nd edition but excluded from this analysis were 45 mesenchymal tumours, 49 malignant lymphomas, 29 metastatic tumours, and 115 tumour-like lesions (sialosis, lymphoepithelial disease, cysts).

Intervention or Treatment Received

Surgery was the primary treatment in most of the neoplasms studied. All benign tumours, apart from PSAs, were treated with surgery (single modality); however, more extended resection in the form of partial maxillectomy was selected in four cases with benign lesions of the minor salivary glands. Primary surgery was the treatment of choice alone or in combination with radium implants for PSAs before 1956. Whenever tumour spillage was noted intraoperatively or in cases that were referred due to residual or recurrent disease, adjuvant radiotherapy (ART) was utilised.

In 244 malignant cases, resection of the primary tumour was mostly followed by ART. Twenty patients were treated by (primary) radical radiotherapy and 27 patients received palliative radiotherapy.

Results

In this study, 950 benign lesions and/or tumours (80%), and 244 malignant SGTs (20%) were included. PSAs accounted for 65% of total tumours, and the parotid glands were most commonly affected (91%). Tumours that were encountered in the submandibular (42%) or minor salivary glands (52%) were more likely to be malignant.

Regarding benign lesions, PSA outnumbered all other lesions combined, followed by adenolymphomas (Warthin's tumour) and monomorphic adenomas. There were nine recurrences in new parotid PSA (1.6%) (median follow-up 12.5 years, with a range of 1–34). There was no recurrence in the 19 patients who received radiation following surgical spillage. No recurrence was recorded in 21 submandibular gland excisions and only 1 following treatment of 22 new PSA in the minor glands. The recurrence rate in patients treated with parotid PSA referred following treatment elsewhere was 15% (median follow-up 14 (range 1–39) years). Malignant degeneration of histologically proven PSA was observed in four patients.

Malignant lesions represented 20% of total tumours. The most common malignancy diagnosis was adenoid cystic carcinoma followed by mucoepidermoid carcinoma (Table 34.1).

The clinical stage and sites of primary malignancies are shown in Table 34.2.

Table 34.1 Distribution of different histological types by anatomical site

	Parotid	Submandibular	Minor	Total
Benign tumours				
Pleomorphic adenoma	721	27	28	776 (65)
Adenolymphoma	159	0	0	159 (13)
Monomorphic adenoma*	12	0	3	15 (1)
Total	892	27	31	950 (80)
Malignant tumours				
Adenoid cystic carcinoma	43	10	22	75 (6)
Mucoepidermoid carcinoma				
Low grade	28	0	7	38 (3)
High grade	3	0	0	
Undifferentiated carcinoma	34	2	2	38 (3)
Adenocarcinoma†	28	2	1	31 (3)
Malignant mixed tumour	21	2	1	24 (2)
Acinic cell carcinoma	20	1	1	22 (2)
Squamous cell carcinoma	13	2	0	15 (1)
Epithelial–myoepithelial carcinoma	0	1	0	1 (0)
Total	190	20	34	244 (20)
Total	1082 (91)	47 (4)	65 (5)	1194 (100)

Values in parentheses are percentages. *Includes oncocytoma and basal cell adenoma; †includes basal cell adenocarcinoma, papillary cystadenocarcinoma, mucinous adenocarcinoma and adenocarcinoma, not otherwise specified.

(Table 2, page 1751: Renehan A, Gleave EN, Hancock BD, Smith, McGurk M. Long-term follow-up over 1000 patients with salivary gland tumours treated in a single centre. Br J Surg 1996;83:1750–4.)

The 5-year, 10-year and 15-year disease-free survival for malignancies that were first treated at this institution ($n = 148$) were 58%, 47% and 45%, respectively, and for recurrent tumours ($n = 61$) were 51%, 43% and 37%, respectively. Recurrences had poorer prognosis than primary tumours, but this was not statistically significant. Seven patients underwent neck dissection; all for parotid malignancies. Locoregional failure rates following treatment of primary carcinoma were parotid, 37% (43/117); submandibular, 5/8; minor glands, 8/23. Distant failure occurred in 24% of newly treated malignancies despite curative intent. Clinically detectable distant metastases were documented in 66 patients (pulmonary 64%; cerebral 24%; skeletal 21%; hepatic 9%).

Table 34.2 Clinical stage (American Joint Committee on Cancer) at initial presentation by anatomical site

Stage	Parotid	Submandibular	Minor
I	32 (24)	0	4
II	37 (27)	3	11
III	25 (18)	2	2
IV	42 (31)	6	4
Total	136 (100)*	11	21*

Values in parentheses are percentages. *There was insufficient clinical information for staging of five parotid and two minor gland carcinomas.

(Table 3, page 1751: Renehan A, Gleave EN, Hancock BD, Smith, McGurk M. Long-term follow-up over 1000 patients with salivary gland tumours treated in a single centre. Br J Surg 1996; 83: 1750–4. John Wiley & Sons.)

The authors divided malignant tumours into three subgroups:

> Group 1 ("good"); low-grade mucoepidermoid carcinoma, acinic cell
> carcinoma, and adenocarcinoma
> Group 2 ("intermediate"); adenoid cystic carcinoma
> Group 3 ("poor"); squamous cell, malignant mixed, high-grade
> mucoepidermoid, and undifferentiated carcinomas.

Group 3 had the worst outcomes. Advanced clinical stage and group 3 tumours
were the strongest prognostic factors of poor outcome on multivariate analysis.

In terms of complications, permanent facial paralysis was less than 3% for benign
lesions, increasing to 36% for malignant tumours. Three deaths were recorded:
one patient died due to meningitis as late sequelae of osteoradionecrosis
following postoperative radiotherapy for parotid malignancy and two patients
died of cardiopulmonary complications immediately after surgery.

Study Limitations

This was a retrospective study reporting quite a heterogeneous cohort of
histological diagnosis and treatment modalities. However, it is admirable that the
authors managed to collect and systematically present coherent, meaningful, and
clinically invaluable data in an era when cancer registries were in their initial stages
of conception and data access through computerised informatics was limited.

The authors acknowledged that definitive histology was established after
surgery. Fine-needle aspiration cytology (FNAC), core biopsy, or MRI scanning
was not routinely available at the time; hence there was limited information
available about the nature of disease preoperatively.

Relevant Studies

There is a lack of prospective randomised trials in this context and overall salivary
gland cancers are uncommon (1–6% of head and neck tumours) and histologically
diverse, which has implications on treatment modalities and outcomes.[2] The
management of benign major SGTs has changed with the advent of extracapsular
dissection (ECD) In a recent review, Brennan et al. reported that ECD is
effective in terms of local control (comparable or even better than superficial
parotidectomy, (SP)) minimising morbidity to the facial nerve (permanent risk
0–1.3% ECD versus 4% SP, temporary risk 8% ECD versus 20% SP).[3]

In relation to the management of recurrent pleomorphic adenoma (RPA), recent
reviews suggest that the risk of RPA is 1–4% for SP and ECD, and 0–1% after
total parotidectomy.[3–5] The rate of second/subsequent RPA increases to 43–45%
following treatment of recurrent tumours. A third RPA tends to present with
multifocal disease.

Most recurrences occur within 7–10 years. Size, histopathological subtype (myxoid), satellite nodules, inadequate encapsulation, and attempted enucleation are risk factors for recurrence. The risk of permanent facial nerve injury after surgery for RPA varies from 11% to 40%. ECD or SP should be offered in patients with solitary and/or localised disease, whereas total parotidectomy is recommended in multifocal disease. ART should be considered in high-risk groups when there is concern for residual disease left in the tumour bed and/or involved resection margins, and when there is no future viable option for surgical salvage without compromising long-term function of the facial nerve, especially the zygomatic branch. Patients unfit for surgery or the elderly group with slowly growing tumours can be considered for palliative radiotherapy if symptomatic, or closely followed up if asymptomatic.

A recent review by Wang et al. addressed the role of radical radiotherapy versus surgery with or without ART.[6] The authors concluded that for early-staged cancers, ART does not add any survival benefit to patients, and that surgery followed by ART offers better outcomes where indicated, for example, tumours larger than 4 cm, high-grade tumours, pN+ve status, and involvement of major nerves or adjacent structures (Tables 34.3 and 34.4).

The risk of occult cervical nodal metastasis depends on several factors: tumour bulk (20% for >4 cm versus 4% <4 cm), tumour grade (Table 34.5) (low 0% versus high 35%), and tumour site (submandibular 42% versus parotid 25%).[6]

For malignant tumours, De Felice et al. recommended greater than 2 cm resection margins for major salivary glands and for adenoid cystic carcinoma in minor salivary glands, and a margin of at least 1 cm in other minor salivary gland

Table 34.3 Management of salivary gland malignancies—adjuvant/postoperative radiotherapy versus primary radiotherapy

Study	Year	Neck Treatment		Treatment	Median Dosage	n	Survival Rate	P
		RT	ND					
Liu et al. [11]	2008	9	–	S+RT	69.7 Gy	10	54.8% (5-year OS)	0.024
				RT	71.4 Gy	10	0%	
Cianchetti et al. [12]	2009	–	21	S+RT	69.6 Gy	76	55% (10-year OS)	0.027
				RT	74.3 Gy	64	35%	
Mendenhall et al. [13]	2005	120	59	S+R	66 Gy	160	48% (10-year OS)	0.0482
				RT	74.0 Gy	64	35%	
Mendenhall et al. [14]	2004	55	13	S+RT	67.8 Gy	59	77% (5-year AS)	NS
				RT	72.4 Gy	42	57%	
Terhaard et al. [15]	2005	120	–	S+RT	62.6 Gy·	386	94% (5-year LC)	<0.0005
					63 Gy	40	50%	
Schramn et al. [16]	2001	–	15	S+RT	52–66 Gy	23	67% (5-year DFS)	NS
Iseli et al. [17]	2009	–	–	S+RT	62.0 Gy	93	75.5% (10-year LRFS)	0.001
				RT	66.0 Gy	10	24.6%	

Abbreviation: n, the number of patients; RT, radiotherapy; S, surgery; OS, overall survival; DFS, disease-free survival; AS, absolute survival; LC, local control; LRFS, local recurrence-free survival; NS, not stated.

Table 34.4 Management of salivary gland malignancies—adjuvant/postoperative radiotherapy versus primary surgery (single modality)

Study	Year	Treatment	Median Dosage	N	Survival Rate	P	LC/RC Rate	p
Armstrong et al. [22]*	1990	PORT	56.6 Gy	46	51% (5-year DS)	0.015	51.3% (5-year LC)	0.14
		S		46	10%		16.8%	
Terhaard et al. [15]	2005	PORT	62.6 Gy	386	NS		91% (10-year LC)	0.0005
		S		112			76%	
Storey et al. [23]	2001	PORT	60.0 Gy	83	NS		88% (5-year LRC)	<0.05
		S		83			50%	
North et al. [24]	1990	PORT	60.0 Gy	50	75% (5-year AS)	0.014	NS (10-year LC)	<0.001
		S		19	59%			
Le et al. [26]	1999	PORT	60.0 Gy	52	63% (10-year OS)	NS	88% (10-year LC)	NS
Terhaard et al. [27]#	2003	PORT	62.0 Gy	385	NS	NS	89% (10-year RC)	0.03
		S		113			67%	

Abbreviation: AS, actuarial survival; DS, determinate survival; LC, local control; LRC, locoregional control; N, the number of patients; NS, not stated; OS, overall survival; PORT, postoperative radiotherapy; RC, regional control; S, surgery.
*, for patients with III and IV disease;#, for N+ patient.

(From Tables 1 & 2, pages 3947–8: Wang X, Luo Y, Li M et al. Management of salivary gland carcinomas—a review. Oncotarget 2017; 8:3946–56. Impact Journals.)

pathologies.[7] This is not always practicable due to the proximity of tumours to vital structures such as the facial nerve. There is a balance therefore between adequacy and practicability when weighing disease survival with function and quality of life outcomes in adopting a personalised approach for patients.

The National Comprehensive Cancer Network guidelines for salivary gland tumours recommends a multidisciplinary approach with head and neck examination, FNA cytology or core biopsy, MRI/CT neck, and CT chest where applicable, along with dental, nutritional, and anaesthetic assessments.[8] There is

Table 34.5 Salivary gland tumour classification based on histology

High Grade	Low Grade
Adenocarcinoma	Low-grade mucoepidermoid carcinoma
High-grade mucoepidermoid carcinoma	Adenoid cystic carcinoma
Salivary duct carcinoma	Polymorphous low-grade Adenocarcinoma
Carcinoma ex pleomorphic adenoma	Basal cell carcinoma
Squamous cell carcinoma	Clear cell carcinoma
Small cell carcinoma	Epithelial-myoepithelial carcinoma
Large cell carcinoma	Sebaceous carcinoma
Carcinosarcoma	Acinic cell carcinoma
Lymphoepithelial carcinoma	
Oncocytic carcinoma	
Myoepithelial carcinoma[2]	

[2] Intermediate/high grade.
(From Table 2, page 96: DeFelice F, deVincentiis M, Valentini V et al. Management of salivary gland malignant tumour: the Policlinico Umberto I, "Sapienza" University of Rome Head and Neck Unit clinical recommendations. Crit Rev Oncol Hematol. 2017;120:93–7. Elsevier.)

level 2A evidence for primary surgery in benign or T1/small T2 tumours, which should be followed by ART in cases of tumour spillage or perineural invasion or adenoid cystic carcinoma pathology. In the management of T3/T4a tumours of major salivary glands or high-risk lesions, neck dissection is recommended for cN0 (and in cN+ve) cases. ART is advisable in patients with adenoid cystic carcinoma, positive margins, perineural and/or lymphovascular invasion, pN+ve, intermediate or high-risk pathology, and pT3/T4 tumours. Radiotherapy should ideally be started ≤6 weeks after surgery and the PTV is 60–66 Gy for high risk, positive margin tumours and 40–55 Gy for low-to-intermediate risk lesions.[7,8]

REFERENCES

1. Gleave EN, Whittaker JS, Nicholson A. Salivary tumours: experience over thirty years. Clin Otolaryngol Allied Sci. 1979; 4: 247–57.
2. Sood S, McGurk M, Vaz F. Management of salivary gland tumours: United Kingdom national multidisciplinary guidelines. J Laryngol Otol. 2016; 130: S142–S9.
3. Brennan PA, Ammar M, Matharu J. Contemporary management of benign parotid tumours: the increasing evidence for extracapsular dissection. Oral Dis. 2017; 23: 18–21.
4. Kanatas A, Ho MWS, Mucke T. Current thinking about the management of recurrent pleomorphic adenoma of the parotid: a structured review. Br J Oral Maxillofac Surg. 2018; 56: 243–8.
5. Witt RL, Nicolai P. Recurrent benign salivary gland neoplasms. Adv Otorhinolaryngol. 2016; 78: 63–70.
6. Wang X, Luo Y, Li M, et al. Management of salivary gland carcinomas: a review. Oncotarget. 2017; 8: 3946–56.
7. De Felice F, de Vincentiis M, Valentini V, et al. Management of salivary gland malignant tumour: the Policlinico Umberto I, "Sapienza" University of Rome head and neck unit clinical recommendations. Crit Rev Oncol Hematol. 2017; 120: 93–7.
8. Pfister D, Spencer S. NCCN Guidelines Version 2.2018 Head and Neck Cancers. 2018.

CHAPTER 35

Capsular Significance in Parotid Tumour Surgery: Reality and Myths of Lateral Lobectomy

Donovan DT, Conley JJ. Laryngoscope. 1984; 94: 324–9.

Reviewed by Toby Pitts-Tucker and Costa Repanos

Research Question/Objective

The current literature suggests that salivary gland tumours account for 3–10% of head and neck neoplasms. Of these 75–85% are parotid in origin. Then, of these 70–80% are benign, with the most common benign tumours being pleomorphic adenomas.[1]

In the early 20th century, surgical enucleation was the mainstay of treatment for all parotid gland tumours. However, this led to high recurrence rates—up to 45% in benign tumours and 90% in high-grade malignant tumours. By the mid-20th century, lateral lobectomy (now also commonly referred to as superficial parotidectomy (SP)) or total parotidectomy with facial nerve dissection and preservation replaced enucleation as the gold standard for the surgical management of parotid tumours. Following this change recurrence rates in benign tumours fell to 2%.[2]

The objective of this study is to explain why a reduction in recurrence rates was seen following this change in surgical practice, and to propose the technique of "capsular dissection" or "limited enucleation" as a viable surgical alternative for benign parotid neoplasms.

Study Design

A retrospective, single-centre case series of parotid gland tumours from the Department of Pathology at the Columbia Presbyterian Medical Centre between 1978 and 1981.

The study reviewed the histological classification of tumours alongside adequacy of surgical margins. Adequacy was defined as the presence of a "cuff of normal parotid tissue surrounding the tumour margins." Further distinction is made between inadequate margins and close margins, which are defined as a 1–2 mm margin or a "thin rim of fibrous tissue only."

Sample Size

A total of 100 consecutive cases were included in this study.

Inclusion/Exclusion Criteria

Only cases of benign mixed tumours or low-grade malignant neoplasms were included. The latter were defined as low-grade muco-epidermoid or acinic cell carcinoma.

Intervention or Treatment Received

All patients underwent lateral lobectomy or total parotidectomy with facial nerve preservation by "currently accepted surgical techniques for parotid tumour management." As the study points out, there is considerable heterogeneity in how these operations were actually performed, owing to the various technical challenges of parotid surgery.

Results

Out of 100 histological samples, 39% had margins which were considered adequate, 40% had close margins, and 21% had tumour extending to the margins.

The authors claim these results demonstrate that lateral lobectomy or total parotidectomy with facial nerve preservation does not represent a pure *en-bloc* resection. Instead, a capsular dissection is inadvertently being performed in the majority (61%) of cases. Thus, it is illusory to think that lateral lobectomy produces a specimen that has the neoplasm in a central position totally surrounded by normal parenchyma.

By correlating these extrapolations with the fall in recurrence rates documented elsewhere in the literature, the authors endorsed capsular dissection as an acceptable surgical approach for benign parotid tumours.

The authors argued that there are some inherent features of the lateral lobectomy, namely its meticulousness and improved exposure, which makes recurrence less likely. However, these features can be transposed to capsular dissection to produce acceptable rates of recurrence according to the authors.

Study Limitations

Examining just 100 cases, this study is not sufficiently powered to make any compelling conclusions about the appropriate surgical approach to parotid tumours. With data drawn from only one centre, there is no evidence to suggest that capsular dissection is inadvertently performed in the majority of lateral lobectomies elsewhere. The study also does not state how many different surgeons were involved in performing these operations. Failure to achieve *en-bloc* resection could, for example, simply be due to the poor surgical technique of just one surgeon.

The data collected is purely histological, and the authors' claims are thus made without any recourse to follow-up data. Pleomorphic adenomas have been known to recur up to 15 years following primary surgery,[3] and this study's failure to address any follow-up seriously diminishes the strength of its conclusions. Also lacking in the results is any mention of preoperative assessment of the parotid tumours, although it does state that "case histories" were examined. This omission is important, as it is the process by which a tumour is deemed to be benign or malignant, a key step in surgical planning.

It is not clear on what basis the authors judge their margins to be "adequate," and although their categorisation appears to be reasonable, there remains no consensus on the adequacy of benign parotid tumour margins.[4]

In a study which proposes capsular dissection as an adequate treatment for benign parotid tumours, incorporation of mortality and morbidity data is markedly absent. What little discussion there is relates only to pre-existing data in the literature. The authors claim that the fall in recurrence rates is largely due to better surgical training and knowledge of pathological processes, and yet no evidence is given to support these claims.

Relevant Studies

The surgical management of benign parotid tumours remains controversial. Parotid gland tumours are rare and have very broad histological heterogeneity, making generation of high-level evidence challenging.

This article sits at the vanguard of research proposing that capsular dissection (now more commonly described as extracapsular dissection, or ECD) is an acceptable alternative to SP for benign parotid tumours. The reasons most commonly cited are that they both have similar rates of recurrence but that ECD has lower rates of complications, particularly in facial nerve injury and Frey's syndrome. The debate is also confused by the complexity of nomenclature for parotid surgery. For example, one study identified nine different terms for SP and five terms for ECD in the literature.[1]

There are no randomised controlled trials for ECD versus SP for benign parotid tumours. The highest level of evidence to inform gold standard surgical treatment is level 2a, in the form of meta-analysis.

Albergotti et al. examined data for 1,882 patients across nine studies, mostly retrospective cohort studies, with a median follow-up of 12 years (range 2–32) (Chapter 36). This concluded that SP should remain the standard of care for treatment of benign parotid tumours, but ECD may be considered by surgeons trained in its application. ECD should, however, be avoided in the presence of any concern for malignancy either preoperatively or intraoperatively.[5]

Foresta et al. pooled data from 19 studies to conclude that for patients with unilateral pleomorphic adenoma within the superficial parotid lobe, with no facial nerve involvement and less than 4 cm in size, ECD is a viable alternative to SP. However, for tumours greater than 4 cm, with poor mobility, malignant histology, or deep lobe involvement, ECD should be avoided. The authors concede that the follow-up was too short to yield a reliable assessment of the recurrence rate though.[1]

The problem with these recommendations is that surgeons cannot always be confident that they are dealing with benign disease preoperatively, even with the benefit of fine-needle aspiration cytology (FNAC). One systematic review of FNAC found the specificity to be 98% for the diagnosis of neoplasia and 96% for malignancy, whereas the sensitivity was 96% for the diagnosis of neoplasia and 79% for the diagnosis of malignancy. There was also significant variation due to reporting expertise.[6] Frozen section pathology may aid diagnosis but is not always available and has its own pitfalls.

Unexpected malignancy following ECD for presumed benign disease also poses fresh challenges for ongoing management. Completion parotidectomy would be a common surgical recommendation, but there is no consensus on the adequacy of margins in redo parotid surgery. Complication rates for redo surgery are also much higher, and it is not clear what role, if any, radiotherapy should play in the management of these patients.

Another problem with surgical approaches to parotid tumours lies in the histological features of the most common benign tumour, pleomorphic adenomas. These lack a complete capsule and often feature microscopic extensions beyond the pseudo-capsule. As a result, recurrence in benign tumours after surgery is relatively common, and due to their indolent growth, recurrence can present late. This is relevant because the preferred treatment for recurrent pleomorphic adenoma is surgery, which is invariably highly challenging given the effects of scarring and the potential for multiple foci of residual disease. Current UK guidelines would suggest a follow-up of 10 years or more for salivary gland neoplasms,[7] but as previously stated, studies comparing SP against ECD often comprise inadequate follow-up to confidently report on recurrence rates. For these reasons in our opinion, SP remains the treatment of choice for parotid gland tumours, even when benign histology is expected.

REFERENCES

1. Foresta E, Torroni A, Di Nardo F, et al. Pleomorphic adenoma and benign parotid tumours: extracapsular dissection vs superficial parotidectomy — review of literature and meta-analysis. Oral Surg Oral Med Oral Pathol Oral Radiol. 2014; 117: 663–76.
2. Donovan D, Conley J. Capsular significance in parotid tumour surgery. Laryngoscope. 1984; 94: 324–9.

3. Dulguerov P, Todic J, Pusztaszeri M, Alotaibi N. Why do parotid pleomorphic adenomas recur? A systematic review of pathological and surgical variables. Front Surg. 2017; 4: 26.
4. Witt R. The significance of the margin in parotid surgery for pleomorphic adenoma. Laryngoscope. 2002; 112: 2141–54.
5. Albergotti W, Nguyen S, Zenk J, Gillespie M. Extracapsular dissection for benign parotid tumours: a meta-analysis. Laryngoscope. 2012; 122: 1954–60.
6. Schmidt R, Hall B, Wilson A, Layfield L. A systematic review and meta-analysis of the diagnostic accuracy of fine-needle aspiration cytology for parotid gland lesions. Am J Clin Pathol. 2011; 136: 45–59.
7. Sood S, McGurk M, Vaz F. Management of salivary gland tumours: United Kingdom national multidisciplinary guidelines. J Laryngol Otol. 2016; 130: S142–9.

CHAPTER 36

Extracapsular Dissection for Benign Parotid Tumours: A Meta-Analysis

Albergotti WG, Nguyen SA, Zenk J, Gillespie MB.
Laryngoscope. 2012; 122: 1954–60.

Reviewed by Konstantinos Mantsopoulos

Research Question/Objective

The aim of this study was to investigate the complication rates and surgical effectiveness (measured as recurrence rate) of extracapsular dissection (ECD) versus superficial parotidectomy (SP) for the treatment of primary benign parotid neoplasms. ECD was defined as the dissection of the tumour with a thin margin of surrounding gland tissue without the intention for identification of the main trunk or branches of the facial nerve. Both complete and partial superficial parotidectomy were defined as superficial parotidectomy, where a portion of or the whole superficial lobe was removed with the tumour after planned identification and dissection of the main trunk and branches of the facial nerve.

Study Design

Systematic literature review with meta-analysis.

Sample Size

Nine articles meeting inclusion criteria identified through an Ovid/Medline search were evaluated in this meta-analysis. The majority of the studies were performed with a retrospective cohort design, although one was prospective. The evaluated studies included a total of 1,882 patients, of which 1,102 underwent ECD and 780 were treated by means of SP. The number of patients in each study included in this meta-analysis varied from 40 to 662, with the percentage of patients who underwent ECD in each study also varying widely, from 2.5% to 75%.

Follow-up

The median follow-up time of the included studies was 12 years, ranging from 2 to 32 years.

Inclusion/Exclusion Criteria

The authors included studies in their meta-analysis that compared ECD to
SP with regard to at least one oncological (tumour recurrence) or functional
(postoperative facial weakness, Frey's syndrome) outcome in the surgical
management of solitary parotid lesions, without suspicion of malignancy on
preoperative clinical and imaging examination. Studies were excluded if they
included recurrent or multiple tumours where the data could not be separated
from primary solitary tumours, tumours of non-parotid origin located in the
parotid gland, or included histologically proven malignant neoplasms. Article
abstracts were reviewed to determine whether the inclusion and exclusion
criteria were fulfilled in each case.

Results

The recurrence rates for ECD and SP were 1.5% (14 of 963 cases) and 2.4% (16
of 670 cases), respectively; statistical analysis could not detect any statistically
significant difference between the compared surgical modalities (OR, 0.557; 95%
CI, 0.271–1.147). There was no difference in follow-up time in most of the studies;
however, two of the articles mentioned a slightly longer follow-up for ECD cases
compared to SP (9 and 10.3 years versus 8 and 8.3 years, respectively). The rate of
transient facial nerve paresis for ECD was 8.0% (59 of 741) and 20.4% (81 of 397)
for SP, demonstrating a mean reduction of 75% in transient facial nerve paresis
for ECD when compared to SP (OR, 0.256; 95% CI, 0.174–0.377). No statistically
significant difference in the rate of permanent facial nerve paralysis between the
two surgical techniques could be detected; interestingly, 1.4% (8 of 590) of ECD
and 1.1% (3 of 268) of SP cases experienced this severe complication (OR, 0.878;
95% CI, 0.282–2.730). Symptomatic Frey's syndrome was reported by 4.5% (27 of
602) of ECD patients compared to 26.1% (75 of 287) of SP patients, which is an
88% reduction in symptomatic Frey's syndrome in the ECD group compared to
the SP group (OR, 0.117; 95% CI, 0.071–0.191).

Study Limitations

The clinical significance of the meta-analysis' results is limited through severe
selection bias as to which surgical modality was performed in each case, as well
as lack of randomisation: It is very likely therefore that patients who underwent
the two methods had different types of tumours in terms of size, palpability and
localisation and that ECD was selectively applied to more manageable (smaller,
palpable, localised caudally) lesions.

An additional limitation of several of the included studies in this meta-analysis
is the reporting of only the oncological and functional results with excision
of pleomorphic adenoma. Recurrence of a pleomorphic adenoma might be
attributed to the surgical technique chosen, to an intraoperative adverse
incident (e.g., intraoperative rupture of the capsule), or surgical error (narrow
resection margins) on the grounds of an undoubtedly demanding lesion from

a histopathologic point of view (incomplete capsule with tumour herniation, pseudopodia, and satellite nodules in up to 20–30%).

On the other hand, recurrence of an ECD-resected cystadenolymphoma is not related to the metachronous appearance of the tumour-like lesion in another site of the parotid gland (10% are known to be multiple). Although pleomorphic adenoma is the pathology most often removed by ECD, it is important to note the recurrence rates and complications for other benign tumours as well as for tumours that were clinically benign but following resection were found to not be benign. Interestingly, it seems that beginning with the "false" working hypothesis and performing less invasive surgery (e.g., ECD) on the ground of an unexpected malignancy appears to be as common as 3–5% of all ECD cases and thus not that particularly rare.

None of the included nine studies explained the diagnostic methodology for evaluating Frey's syndrome. Furthermore, insufficient detail was provided on the timing of seeking for and evaluating of this specific complication, which may be relevant because symptomatic Frey's syndrome in the immediate postoperative period may lessen over time and not be detectable in the long term.

Relevant Studies

Extracapsular dissection (ECD) in its current form (dissection around the tumour capsule with a cuff of healthy tissue around it using facial nerve monitoring, without intending to expose the facial nerve) has been performed for almost 30 years.[1] Before 1990 and in the first half of the 20th century, the surgical concepts of intracapsular enucleation (opening the capsule of the tumour and "scraping out" the lesion) as well as extracapsular enucleation (dissecting along the tumour capsule) prevailed.[2] Due to the unacceptably frequent recurrences of pleomorphic adenomas as well as malignant tumours, this principle was abandoned and replaced by the philosophy of obligate facial nerve dissection, leading to at least a superficial parotidectomy in each case. The high rate of postoperative facial nerve palsy led to attempts for reduction of surgical invasiveness in the parotid surgery, balancing out today at the level of ECD as a surgically acceptable minimum, with the concept of a minimally invasive but still oncologically safe procedure.[3] This kind of surgery can therefore be considered for single, mobile lesions with preoperative clinical and imaging features of a benign tumour within the superficial lobe of the parotid gland. It may also be an option for multifocal cystadenolymphomas in the tail of the parotid gland as well, and in carefully selected tumours in the deep lobe of the parotid. Conforming to the model of personalised medicine and minimal invasive surgery, this surgical modality, in contrast to superficial parotidectomy, is not defined from the facial nerve as a landmark but is indicated on the basis of the individual clinical and imaging tumour-related characteristics.

In accordance with several other studies[4–6] and considering the previously mentioned study limitations, this meta-analysis shows that a shift towards less-invasive surgical procedures (such as ECD) does not lead to compromises in patient safety, functional outcomes, or postoperative surgical complications.[6,7] In this context, it should be clear that the choice of surgical approach can often be made in the operating room.

ECD is a simple procedure (from a technical point of view) but in terms of defining proper indications is also an advanced treatment modality,[8] and can be very demanding intraoperatively.[9] An increase in extracapsular surgery should be considered to be the result of growing expertise[9] rather than an attempt to save operative time and costs and should be performed by surgeons who are able to recognise and dissect the facial nerve if required.[3]

REFERENCES

1. Renehan A, Gleave EN, Hancock BD, Smith P, McGurk M. Long-term follow-up of over 1000 patients with salivary gland tumours treated in a single centre. Br J Surg. 1996; 83: 1750–4.
2. Rawson AJ, Howard JM, Royster HP, Horn RCJ. Tumours of the salivary glands; A clinicopathological study of 160 cases. Cancer. 1950; 3: 445–58.
3. Mantsopoulos K, Koch M, Klintworth N, Zenk J, Iro H. Evolution and changing trends in surgery for benign parotid tumours. Laryngoscope. 2015; 125: 122–7.
4. George KS, McGurk M. Extracapsular dissection–minimal resection for benign parotid tumours. Br J Oral Maxillofac Surg. 2011; 49: 451–4.
5. Xie S, Wang K, Xu H, et al. PRISMA-extracapsular dissection versus superficial parotidectomy in treatment of benign parotid tumours: evidence from 3194 patients. Medicine (Baltimore). 2015; 94: e1237.
6. Kato MG, Erkul E, Nguyen SA, et al. Extracapsular dissection vs superficial parotidectomy of benign parotid lesions: surgical outcomes and cost-effectiveness analysis. J Am Med Assoc. Otolaryngol Head Neck Surg. 2017; 143: 1092–7.
7. Dell'Aversana Orabona G, Bonavolonta P, Iaconetta G, Forte R, Califano L. Surgical management of benign tumours of the parotid gland: extracapsular dissection versus superficial parotidectomy–our experience in 232 cases. J Oral Maxillofac Surg. 2013; 71: 410–3.
8. Mantsopoulos K, Scherl C, Iro H. Investigation of arguments against properly indicated extracapsular dissection in the parotid gland. Head Neck. 2017; 39: 498–502.
9. Larian B. Parotidectomy for benign parotid tumours. Otolaryngol Clin North Am. 2016; 49: 395–413.

CHAPTER **37**

Excision Margins in High-Risk Malignant Melanoma

Thomas JM, Newton-Bishop J, A'Hern R, et al.
New Eng J Med. 2004; 350: 757–66.

Reviewed by Elizabeth A Gruber

Research Question/Objective

Controversy exists concerning the necessary margin of excision for cutaneous melanoma 2 mm or greater in thickness. This study investigated the effect of excision margin on the outcome of patients with high-risk malignant melanoma.

Study Design

A prospective, multicentre, randomised clinical trial comparing 1 cm and 3 cm excision margins.

Sample Size

A total of 900 patients were recruited. Of these, 453 were randomly assigned to undergo surgery with a 1 cm excision margin and 447 to 3 cm margin of excision.

Follow-up

Time to locoregional recurrence and disease-free survival were the primary endpoints. Overall survival was a secondary endpoint.

Inclusion/Exclusion Criteria

Eligible patients had a single, primary, localised cutaneous melanoma 2 mm or greater in thickness on the trunk or limbs (palms of hands and soles of feet were excluded) where a 3 cm excision margin was technically possible. Patients had to be at least 18 years old and not pregnant. Patients with a history of cancer (other than basal cell carcinoma) or who were receiving immunosuppressive therapy were excluded. Elective lymph node dissection, sentinel node biopsy, or adjuvant therapy were not allowed.

Intervention or Treatment Received

Participating surgeons chose one of two primary approaches. The primary tumour could be excised before randomisation, with either a 1 mm or a 1 cm margin to confirm the diagnosis and determine the thickness of the lesion. Patients were then randomly assigned to receive a 1 cm or 3 cm margin if they had 1 mm primary excision or to receive no further additional treatment or an additional 2 cm margin after the 1 cm primary excision. The trial surgery was required to be performed within 45 days after the primary excision, and all excisions were to extend to or include the deep fascia.

Results

The median tumour thickness was 3.0 mm in the group with 1 cm margin of excision and 3.1 mm in the group with 3 cm margin of excision. The site of melanoma had the expected gender distribution. Among the men, 48.1% had tumours on the back and 18.1% had lower limb tumours, whereas in women 18.4% were on the back and 52.9% on the lower limb. Median follow-up was 60 months.

A 1 cm margin of excision was associated with a significantly increased risk of locoregional recurrence. There were 168 locoregional recurrences (as first events) in the group with 1 cm excision margins, compared with 142 in the group with 3 cm margins (HR, 1.26; 95% CI, 1.00–1.59; $P = 0.05$). There were 128 deaths attributable to melanoma in the group with 1 cm margins, as compared with 105 in the group with 3 cm margins (HR, 1.24; 95% CI, 0.96–1.61; $P = 0.1$). Overall survival was similar in the two groups (HR for death, 1.07; 95% CI, 0.85–1.36; $P = 0.6$).

The rate of surgical complications was 7.8% among patients who had a 1 cm excision margin and 13.9% with a 3 cm margin ($P = 0.05$).

The findings of this study suggest that in a small number of patients the melanoma cells that remain after excision with a 1 cm margin will prove fatal. The authors therefore recommend that the use of 1 cm excision margins should be avoided in patients with melanomas that are 2 mm thick or more.

Study Limitations

The results state there were protocol deviations in 14.0% of patients. These included tumour thickness less than 2 mm on review and 3 cm margin not possible due to site of tumour. Although the authors state that the majority of protocol deviations were minor and they are similar in both groups, this could have affected the results.

Another limitation is that this study did not include patients with head and neck melanoma. This potentially has a different pattern of spread due to the complex anatomy in this region and the facial skin being very thin in some areas. Often more complex reconstruction is required to restore form and function, with the potential for increased morbidity and complications.

Relevant Studies

Wide local excision is the most effective treatment for primary cutaneous melanoma, but the optimal width of excision margins has been contentious. Current treatment guidelines are based on a small number of prospective randomised trials, including this one.[1-3]

The authors of this study provide an overview of excision margin trials, which suggest a significant increase in the risk of death from melanoma associated with a narrow margin of excision, as compared with a wide margin (HR, 1.26; 95% CI, 1.06–1.50; $P = 0.008$). This evidence suggests that wider margins of excision may improve survival in a proportion of patients.[2,4]

National and International Guidelines support the use of wider margins as recommended by relevant studies.

The British Association of Dermatology UK Guidelines (2010) recommend a 2–3 cm surgical excision margin for melanomas over 2 mm up to 4 mm thick.[5] However, the final decision about the size of margin should be made by the MDT after discussion with the patient. The recommendation should be made with consideration of functional and cosmetic implications of the chosen margin.

The NICE Guideline (NG14) July 2015 recommends offering excision with a clinical margin of at least 1 cm to people with Stage I melanoma and at least 2 cm to people with Stage II melanoma.[6]

The 2016 UK National Multidisciplinary Guidelines suggest primary cutaneous invasive melanoma should be excised with a surgical margin of at least 1 cm with a maximum recommended margin of 3 cm. The actual margin of excision depends upon the depth and its anatomical site. For lesions 2.1–4 mm thick, 2–3 cm margins are recommended (2 cm preferred) and for lesions thicker than 4 mm, the recommendation is 2–3 cm.[7] They state that in the head and neck region, anatomical restrictions and cosmetic considerations may preclude even a 1 cm margin. However, in these circumstances the width of excision should remain uniform all the way around the lesion.

The updated ESMO Clinical Practice Guidelines (2019) on cutaneous melanoma recommend wide local excision of 1 cm for tumours with a thickness of up to 2 mm and 2 cm for thicker tumours.[8] It suggests that modifications, with reduced safety margins, are acceptable for preservation of function in acral and facial melanomas and can be performed with the slow Mohs technique, although prospective randomised trials are not available.

The head and neck is an anatomically sensitive area and few papers are specific to this site. The evidence for excision margins is extrapolated from studies on melanoma of other anatomical sites. Outcomes associated with cutaneous head and neck melanoma are poorer when compared with all other sites, with a higher rate of recurrence, shorter disease-free survival, and overall survival.[9] Patient survival is dependent on age, depth of tumour invasion, and histology. A recent population-based cohort analysis of patients with head and neck cutaneous melanoma showed that a wider resection margin (greater than 2 cm) did not confer any additional survival benefit compared with a narrower margin (between 1 and 2 cm).[10] This was the case for lip, scalp, neck, external ear, eyelid, and face. Additionally, the use of wider margins did not confer any survival benefit to patients with more advanced disease, for example, sentinel lymph node spread. These findings are supported by another retrospective study in head and neck melanoma, which shows that distance of histopathological margins does not affect survival.[11]

The NCCN Clinical Practice Guidelines state that surgical margins may be modified to accommodate individual anatomical or functional considerations.[12] A recent retrospective study of 79 patients with head and neck cutaneous melanoma found that local recurrence rates were comparable between reduced margins (to preserve critical anatomical areas such as eyelid, nose, mouth, and auricle) and recommended wide local excision margins.[13] Further prospective studies specific to the head and neck are required.

Mohs micrographic surgery may also have a role, especially on the face.[14] There is growing evidence for its efficacy, but further studies are required before firm recommendations can be made. Frozen section with the addition of immunostaining is also currently under investigation.

REFERENCES

1. Meirion Thomas J, Newton-Bishop J, A'Hern R, et al. Excision margins in high-risk malignant melanoma. N Engl J Med. 2004; 350; 8: 757–66.
2. Cohn-Cedermark G, Rutqvist LE, Andersson R, et al. Long-term results of a randomized study by the Swedish melanoma study group on 2 cm versus 5 cm resection margins for patients with cutaneous melanoma with a tumour thickness of 0.8-2.0 mm. Cancer. 2000; 89: 1495–501.
3. Gillgren P, Drzewiecki KT, Niin M, et al. 2 cm versus 4 cm surgical excision margins for primary cutaneous melanoma thicker than 2 mm: a randomised, multicentre trial. Lancet. 2011; 378: 1635–42.
4. Balch CM, Soong SJ, Smith T, et al. Long-term results of a prospective surgical trial comparing 2 cm vs. 4 cm excision margins for 740 patients with 1-4 mm melanomas. Ann Surg Oncol. 2001; 8: 101–8.
5. Marsden JR, Newton-Bishop JA, Burrows L, et al. Revised U.K. guidelines. Br J Dermatol. 2010; 163: 238–56.
6. NICE Guideline (NG14) July 2015. Available at: https://www.nice.org.uk/guidance/ng14.
7. Ahmed OA, Kelly C. Head and neck melanoma (excluding ocular melanoma): United Kingdom National Multidisciplinary Guidelines. J Laryngol Otol. 2016; 130: S133–S41.

8. Michielin O, van Akkooi A, Ascierto P, Dummer R, Keilholz U. Cutaneous melanoma: ESMO clinical practice guidelines. Ann Oncol. 2019; 30: 1884–901.

9. Fadaki N, Li R, Parrett B. Is head and neck melanoma different from trunk and extremity melanomas with respect to sentinel lymph node status and clinical outcome? Ann Surg Oncol. 2013; 20: 3089–97.

10. Han AY, Dhanjani S, Pettijohn K, Patel PB, St John MA. Optimal resection margin for head and neck cutaneous melanoma. Laryngoscope. 2019; 129: 1386–94.

11. Teng J, Halbert T, McMurry TL, Levine PA, Christophel JJ. Histopathologic margin distance in survival in resection of cutaneous melanoma of the head and neck. Laryngoscope. 2015; 125: 1856–60.

12. National Comprehensive Cancer Network. Practice guidelines in oncology: melanoma. Available at: www.nccn.org.

13. Rawlani R, Rawlani V, Qureshi H. Reducing margins of wide local excision in head and neck melanoma for function and cosmesis: 5 year local recurrence free survival. J Surg Oncol. 2015; 111: 795–9.

14. Whalen J, Leone D. Mohs micrographic surgery for the treatment of malignant melanoma. Clin Dermatol. 2009; 27: 597–602.

CHAPTER 38

Multiprofessional Guidelines for the Management of the Patient with Primary Cutaneous Squamous Cell Carcinoma

Motley R, Kersey P, Lawrence C. Br J Dermatol. 2002; 146: 18–25.

Reviewed by Tatiana Welsch and Lisa Greaney

Summary of Paper

Clinical Presentation and Incidence of cSCC

Cutaneous squamous cell carcinoma (cSCC) is the second most common skin cancer and is a malignant tumour arising from the keratinising cells of the epidermis or its appendages. It accounts for 20% of all cutaneous skin malignancies in the United Kingdom and epidemiologic studies demonstrate a rising incidence worldwide. The UK incidence of cSCC is similarly rising, with a conservative estimated increase of 30% in the last decade.[1] The majority of cases have a good prognosis, but occasionally cSCC will metastasise to regional lymph nodes and distant sites, and accordingly, the potential aggressive nature of this tumour should not be underestimated.

Aetiology of cSCC

A well-established relationship exists between cSCC and chronic cumulative exposure to ultraviolet (UV) radiation, particularly UVB. cSCC most often arises from precursor lesions such as actinic keratosis and SCC in situ (Bowen's disease) but can also develop de novo on chronically inflamed skin and within wounds, burns, and scars or secondary to exposure to ionising radiation (PUVA treatment, indoor tanning devices). Arsenic exposure and the human papilloma virus (types 6, 11, and 16) have also been identified as risk factors. Organ transplant patient (OTP) recipients have a 65–250 times greater risk of cSCC compared to the general population, and in such patients the lesions tend to be more aggressive in nature.[2] This increased incidence of cSCC is thought to be related to immunosuppressive medications.

Diagnosis

Patients with a suspected diagnosis of squamous cell carcinoma should be referred to a dermatology department. The diagnosis of cSCC is established by biopsy or excision and subsequent histological examination. The histology report should comment on the following:

- Degree of differentiation (well, moderately, poorly, or undifferentiated)
- Subtype (verrucous, desmoplastic, spindle, or acantholytic)
- Tumour thickness
- Level of dermal invasion (Clark level)
- Presence or absence of perineural, perivascular, or perilymphatic invasion
- Peripheral and deep margins

Prognosis

According to research, the rate of nodal metastasis of cSCC has been estimated to range from 2% to 5% and disease specific death to be 2.1%.[3]

Factors such as tumour diameter greater than 20 mm, tumour thickness greater than 4 mm, location on the ear, lips, and non-UVR exposed sites such as sacrum or sole of foot, and poor differentiation are indicators of increased risk of metastasis. Perineural invasion (PNI) is associated with an increased risk of tumour recurrence, lymph node metastasis, distant metastasis, and death.

These high-risk cSCCs require multidisciplinary input.

cSCC types derived from invasive Bowen's disease, and cSCCs arising in radiation or thermal scars and ulcers tend to exhibit more aggressive behaviour and have a higher risk of metastasis. Recurrence is more common in lesions at least 4 mm thick that extend to the deep dermis and in patients with underlying immune dysfunction.

Staging

The American Joint Committee for Cancer (AJCC) and the Union for International Cancer Control (UICC) have included a cSCC TNM staging system for head and neck in their 8th editions. The AJCC 8th edition stages the tumour based on diameter, depth of invasion, and presence of PNI. This latter staging system does not, however, apply to non-head and neck cSCCs.

High-stage tumours should be considered for additional imaging and diagnostic evaluation at the time of diagnosis.

Treatment

Surgical Excision

The gold standard of treatment for invasive cSCC consists of complete, histologically confirmed surgical excision of the primary tumour and of any metastases. Surgical excision and Mohs micrographic surgery (MMS) are regarded as the treatment of choice for cutaneous SCC, as they provide tissue for histological examination that allows both the pathologist to assess the adequacy of treatment and the treating physician to undertake further surgery if necessary.

For low-risk tumours, excision with a 4 mm margin is recommended, whereas margins of at least 6 mm are recommended for high-risk tumours. Brodland et al. published a study which showed that obtaining a 4 mm margin for lesions with a diameter of 2 cm or less would result in a 95% negative margin rate, and a 6 mm margin for lesions with a diameter greater than 2 cm would achieve the equivalent negative margin rate.[4] This can be difficult to achieve in certain anatomical areas and may result in cosmetic and functional impairment.

Lansbury et al. undertook a systematic review of 12 observational studies, and the rate of local recurrence following surgical removal of invasive cSCCs in 1,144 patients ranged from 0% to 15% with a pooled average rate of 5.4%.[5]

Van Lee et al. published a retrospective cohort study comparing the risk of recurrence between MMS and standard excision for cSCC of the head and neck.[4] A total of 579 patients with 672 cSCCs were included: 380 were treated with MMS and 292 with standard excision. The risk of recurrence was 8% after standard excision during a median follow-up of 5–7 years, which was higher than the 3% after MMS during a median follow-up of 4–9 years. The cumulative incidence of recurrence was higher for standard excision than for MMS during the entire follow-up period of 8.6 years. Carcinomas treated with MMS had a three times lower risk of recurrence than those treated with standard excision when adjusted for tumour size and deep tumour invasion (adjusted HR 0·31; 95% CI, 0·12–0·66).

A systematic review by Lansbury et al. of 2,133 MMS-treated cSCCs removed from all anatomical sites found a resultant pooled cure rate of 97.4% (95%CI, 96.2%–98.3%. MMS aims to preserve as much normal tissue as possible. Therefore, where wide surgical margins may result in functional and cosmetic impairment, MMS should be considered the preferred treatment choice.[6]

Radiotherapy

Radiotherapy is a valid treatment option for cSCCs where surgical excision is not possible without functional or cosmetic impairment. A systematic review by Lansbury et al. of 761 patients who underwent primary radiation for cSCCs found a local recurrence rate of 6.4% (95% CI, 3.0–11.0%) and death from disease of 9.1% (95% CI, 1.4–22.8%).[6]

Primary radiotherapy requires the involvement of a qualified clinical oncologist. In all cases where there is debate about whether radiotherapy or surgery is the best option, close liaison should take place between the dermatologist, clinical oncologist and maxillofacial/plastic surgeon, ideally in a multidisciplinary clinic.

Adjuvant radiotherapy is currently recommended for cSCC cases with large caliber nerve invasion (>0.1 mm nerve diameter), cases with uncertain or positive surgical margins, or as salvage treatment for cases not treated with surgery or those with in-transit metastasis.

Chemoprophylaxis

Nicontinamide is the amide form of vitamin B3, and a phase III randomised controlled trial (RCT) of nicotinamide 500 mg twice a day compared to placebo found a 23% reduction in the rate of new non-melanoma skin cancer development in the nicotinamide group compared to placebo group ($P = 0.02$). In addition, the risk of new cSCC development in nicotinamide group was reduced by 30% ($P = 0.05$) during a 12-month period.[7]

Multidisciplinary Review

Patients with high-risk SCC and those presenting with clinically involved lymph nodes should be reviewed by a multiprofessional skin oncology team, which includes a dermatologist, pathologist, appropriately trained surgeon (usually a plastic, ENT or maxillofacial surgeon), clinical oncologist, radiologist, and clinical nurse specialist in skin cancer.

Follow-up

Seventy-five percent of local recurrences and metastases are detected within 2 years and 95% within 5 years. It would therefore seem reasonable for the patient who has had a high-risk SCC to be kept under close medical observation for recurrent disease for at least 2 and up to 5 years. The patient should receive adequate information about the tumour and about how to self-examine his or her lymph nodes. Sun avoidance, the use of protective clothing and effective sunblocks should be promoted.

Importance to Modern Practice and Further Relevant Papers

Since the original 2002 paper, the British Association of Dermatologists (BAD) has updated its guidelines in 2009 and SIGN published further guidelines in 2017. The latest changes include curtailing high-risk sites (e.g., external ear, PNI, two histological subtypes), but the majority of recommendations remain as per original guidelines discussed previously.

Conclusion

The incidence of cSCC continues to rise worldwide. Upon review of the multiprofessional guidelines originally published in 2002, current therapeutic strategies remain mostly unchanged. While cSCC generally carries a good prognosis, the risk of metastasis does exist in patients with high risk subtypes and such patients require close monitoring. Early diagnosis and prevention of cSCC remain key elements of the management approach.

REFERENCES

1. Toby GN, Richard EA. Low incidence of metastasis and recurrence from cutaneous squamous cell carcinoma found in a UK population: do we need to adjust our thinking on this rare but potentially fatal event? J Surg Oncol. 2017; 116: 783–8.
2. Soodeh K, Chrysalyne DS, Emily SR. A review of cutaneous squamous cell carcinoma epidemiology, diagnosis, and management. Int J Cancer Manag. 2018; 11: e60846.
3. Stratigos AJ, Garbe C, Dessinioti C, et al. European Dermatology Forum (EDF), the European Association of Dermato-Oncology (EADO) and the European Organization for Research and Treatment of Cancer (EORTC). European interdisciplinary guideline on invasive squamous cell carcinoma of the skin: Part 1. epidemiology, diagnostics and prevention. Eur J Cancer. 2020; 128: 60–82.
4. Brodland DG, Zitelli JA. Surgical margins for excision of primary cutaneous squamous cell carcinoma. J Am Acad Dermatol. 1992; 27: 241–8.
5. Lansbury L, Bath-Hextall F, Perkins W, Stanton W, Leonardi-Bee J. Interventions for non-metastatic squamous cell carcinoma of the skin: systematic review and pooled analysis of observational studies. Br Med J. 2013; 347: f6153.
6. van Lee CB, Roorda BM, Wakkee M, et al. Recurrence rates of cutaneous squamous cell carcinoma of the head and neck after Mohs micrographic surgery vs. standard excision: a retrospective cohort study. Br J Dermatol. 2019; 181: 338–43.
7. Chen AC, Martin AJ, Choy B, et al. A phase 3 randomized trial of nicotinamide for skin-cancer chemoprevention. N Engl J Med. 2015; 373: 1618–26.

Final Trial Report of Sentinel-Node Biopsy versus Nodal Observation in Melanoma

Morton DL, Thompson JF, Cochran AJ, et al. N Engl J Med. 2014; 370: 599–609.

Reviewed by Peter T Glen and Daryl Godden

Research Question

Does sentinel lymph node biopsy (SLNB) in the management of cutaneous melanoma confer a survival advantage?

Ever since Snow advocated elective nodal dissection (END) in 1892,[1] the management of the draining nodal basin has been contentious. The central concept for SLNB to work is that there must be contiguous spread to lymph nodes before distant metastasis ensues. Unfortunately, large randomised trials showed that overall there was no survival advantage following END although some subsets of patients had a small improvement.[2–4] END has a high risk of complications including limb lymphoedema and consequently there was a move away from END as the technique of SLNB was developed. This aimed to offer a survival advantage by early treatment of clinically negative metastases with reduced morbidity.

Study Design

This was a multicentre randomised controlled trial in which patients were randomised to either SLNB and subsequent completion lymphadenectomy if positive, or observation and therapeutic dissection if disease became apparent. The patients were followed up for 10 years. The endpoint was melanoma-specific survival.

Sample Size

A total of 2,001 patients were recruited into the study, and 1,347 patients with intermediate thickness melanoma (1.2–3.5 mm) were identified. There were 340 patients with thin melanoma (1.0–1.2 mm) and 314 patients with thick melanoma (greater than 3.5 mm).

Follow-up

Patients were monitored postoperatively by means of clinical examination, blood testing, and chest radiography every 3 months for 2 years, every 4 months in year 3, every 6 months in years 4 and 5, and annually after 5 completed years. Participating sites used their own protocols, which could include computed tomography (CT) or positron emission tomography-computed tomography (PET-CT), nodal ultrasound, S100, and lactate dehydrogenase (LDH) serology.

Inclusion/Exclusion Criteria

The criteria for enrollment included patients with localised cutaneous melanoma, Clark level 3, or Breslow thickness of 1.00 mm or more. Patients were aged between 18 and 75 years of age and had to have an anticipated survival of 10 years or more at recruitment.[5]

Exclusion criteria included patients who had had a 3 cm excision and tumour clearance was 1.5 cm or more. Patients with satellites, in-transit metastases, regional, or distant disease were excluded. Full details can be found at the Multicentre Selective Lymphadenectomy Trial (MSLT).[5]

Intervention

Eligible patients were randomly assigned to wide excision of the primary melanoma plus SLNB or wide excision alone and observation. For intermediate thickness melanoma a 2–3 cm margin was recommended.

Sentinel nodes from the SLNB group were investigated with hematoxylin and eosin, S100, HMB 45, and MelanA. The presence of immunopositive nodes even in a single cell was counted as positive and the patients underwent a completion lymphadenectomy.

Patients in the observation group would undergo therapeutic lymphadenectomy if nodes became clinically apparent.

Results

A total of 1,270 patients in the intermediate thickness group could be evaluated (770 had SLNB and 500 observation). There were 290 patients with thick melanoma and 232 with thin melanoma.

For intermediate thickness melanoma, there was no overall melanoma specific survival at 10 years for the SLNB Test Group when compared to the Observation Group with mean (+/-SE) rates of 81.4 +/− 1.5% vs. 78.3 +/− 2.0% respectively (hazard ratio for death from melanoma in the biopsy group, 0.84; 95% confidence interval [CI], 0.64–1.09; $P = 0.18$).

The 10-year melanoma-specific survival in the SNLB Test Group who were node negative was no different to that of the Observation Group (88.0 +/− 1.4% vs. 86.6 +/− 1.8%).

The 10-year disease-specific survival for the SLNB Test Group who were node positive was 62.1 +/− 4.8%; this compared to 41.5 +/− 5.6% in the Observation Group who developed nodal disease. Thus, SNLB demonstrated a 20% survival advantage in node-positive patients compared to the Observation Group who developed nodes.

Initially, the rate of detection of positive nodes following SNLB was 16%; however, during follow-up 4.8% of SNLB-negative patients developed disease in their draining lymph nodes, resulting in a false-negative rate of 4.8% and a sensitivity of 80%.

Study Limitations

This is the only large multicentre randomised controlled study investigating SNLB in cutaneous melanoma. Its aim was to establish whether SNLB confers a survival advantage. In the interim report,[6] it was evident that there was no difference in melanoma-specific survival and the authors subsequently undertook a subset analysis. Their post hoc data showed an improvement in survival in SNLB-positive patients when compared to the therapeutic nodal dissection patients in the Observation Group. This post hoc analysis was widely criticised at the time.

The false-positive rate of 4.8% (and consequent 80% sensitivity) was explained by the authors, who pointed out that initially SNLB was technique sensitive and there was a learning curve as it became more widely adopted. The authors also explained that initially blue dye (patent blue) was used, but sensitivity improved when isotope and single photon emission computed tomography (SPECT) techniques were adopted. The exclusion criteria excluded patients whose melanoma was greater than 1.5 cm from the margin of the melanoma. This is because the lymphatic drainage changes as the distance from the melanoma increases. Today, it is accepted that isotope should be injected 2 mm from the tumour and in consequence, primary excision should be with a 2-mm margin.

Finally, the follow-up of patients was not universal between centres, with chest radiographs, ultrasound, CT, or PET-CT used based on the individual centre's practice.

Relevant Studies

Following this key study, subsequent research has investigated the need for a completion lymphadenectomy. Faries et al. in MSLT-II demonstrated that there was no survival advantage in a randomised controlled trial of completion lymphadenectomy compared to observation.[7] Only 11.5% of patients were found to have non-sentinel nodal metastases following dissection.

DeCOG-SLT is a large multicentre trial on completion lymphadenectomy versus observation in patients with SLNB positive melanoma. Researchers found no significant survival benefit between the two groups and subsequently recommended observation only for micrometastases of 1 mm or less, avoiding the need for a completion lymphadenectomy.[8] However, the Melanoma Focus multidisciplinary consensus meeting held in 2018 recently published guidelines advising that completion lymphadenectomy should be considered where there is a high risk of relapse: extracapsular spread, more than three sentinel nodes, and multifocal or extensive disease where adjuvant therapy is not possible or available.[9]

With the advent of biologics and immunotherapy we have better ways of treating SNLB-positive patients[10,11], and in the future SLNB will not only offer prognostic information, it will be a key investigation prior to the start of systemic therapies in resected disease.

REFERENCES

1. Snow H. Melanotic cancerous disease. Lancet. 1892; 2: 872–4.
2. Veronesi U, Adamus J, Bandiera DC, et al. Inefficacy of immediate node dissection in stage 1 melanoma of the limbs. N Engl J Med. 1977; 297: 627–30.
3. Cascinelli N, Morabito A, Santinami M, MacKie RM, Belli F. Immediate or delayed dissection of regional nodes in patients with melanoma of the trunk: a randomised trial. Lancet. 1998; 351: 793–6.
4. Balch CM, Soong S, Ross MI, et al. Long-term results of a multi-institutional randomised trial comparing prognostic factors and surgical results for intermediate thickness melanomas (1.0 to 4.0 mm). Ann Surg Oncol. 2000; 7: 87–9.
5. Morton DL, Thompson JF, Cochran AJ, et al. MSLT Group. Final trial report of sentinel-node biopsy versus nodal observation in melanoma. N Engl J Med. 2014; 370: 599–609.
6. Morton DL, Thompson JF, Cochran AJ, et al. MSLT Group. Sentinel-node biopsy or nodal observation in melanoma. N Engl J Med. 2006; 355: 1307–17. Erratum in: N Engl J Med. 2006; 355: 1944.
7. Faries MB, Thompson JF, Cochran AJ, et al. Completion dissection or observation for sentinel-node metastasis in melanoma. N Engl J Med. 2017; 376: 2211–22.
8. Leiter U, Stadler R, Mauch C, et al. Complete lymph node dissection versus no dissection in patients with sentinel lymph node biopsy positive melanoma (DeCOG-SLT): a multicentre, randomised, phase 3 trial. Lancet Oncol. 2016; 17: 757–67.

9. Melanoma Focus. Sentinel node biopsy guideline, based on a multi-disciplinary consensus meeting held 17th May 2018; Cambridge, UK. [Published 3rd Dec 2018–Accessed 4th Dec 2018]. Available from: https://melanomafocus.com/wp-content/uploads/2018/12/SNB-Consensus-Guideline.pdf.

10. Weber J, Mandala M, Del Vecchio M, et al. Adjuvant Nivolumab versus Ipilimumab in resected stage III or IV melanoma. N Engl J Med. 2017; 377: 1824–35.

11. Long GV, Hauschild A, Santinami M, et al. Adjuvant Dabrafenib plus Trametinib in Stage III BRAF-mutated melanoma. N Engl J Med. 2017; 377: 1813–23.

CHAPTER 40

Internal Derangements of the Temporomandibular Joint, Pathological Variations

Wilkes CH. Arch Otolaryngol Head Neck Surg. 1989; 115: 469–77.

Reviewed by Carrol P Saridin and Pieter G Raijmakers

Research Question/Objective

The main objective of this study was to determine the pathological variations, pathophysiology, course, and probable cause of internal derangement of the temporomandibular joint (TMJ).

Study Design

A retrospective analysis of patients who had surgery for internal derangements (ID) of the TMJ over a 15-year period. Patients were derived from a much larger population of patients with TMJ disorders.

Sample Size

A total of 540 operated cases (740 joints) were retrospectively analysed. Pathological analysis of submitted tissue was performed in a subpopulation of 100 consecutive joints.

Follow-up

Not applicable.

Inclusion/Exclusion Criteria

The inclusion criteria were not described apart from having undergone surgery. Unrelated craniofacial pain disorders were excluded on the basis of clinical evaluation and appropriate radiologic and/or laboratory studies.

Intervention or Treatment Received

This is a descriptive study, rather than an effectiveness study of a specific treatment. The preoperative evaluation consisted of tomographic and arthrographic studies and magnetic resonance imaging (MRI) in a subgroup of the population. Radiologic and pathological findings were correlated, and a pathological and time-dependent categorisation was employed to correlate and classify clinical, radiologic, and pathological findings into five groups: early, early/intermediate, intermediate, intermediate/late, and late.

Results

The basic lesion observed was malposition (anterior displacement) and altered structure of the articular disc. There was a near 100% correlation between the presence of disc displacement and the presence of clinical signs and symptoms.

The early stage cases were characterised by painless clicking and a slightly anteriorly displaced disc. The early/intermediate stage had more intense joint sounds, some pain, and occasional locking. As the degenerative process progresses and the disc becomes deformed and blocks condylar movement, there is increased pain and locking, which is the intermediate stage. In the intermediate/late stage, there is increasing deformity of the disc and degenerative changes of the condylar head, which is characterised by a chronic closed lock and joint sounds disappearing. Finally, in the late-stage there is crepitus, pain, and restricted motion of the condyle due to disc perforation, muscle spasm and/or fibrous ankylosis.

The average duration of symptoms was 6.7 years, with a wide range (50% 2–4 years and 25% longer than 10 years). Almost all patients (97%) presented with either intermediate, intermediate/late, or late-stage disease, although this may reflect the study population being patients who had undergone surgery, which would be expected to be restricted to those with more symptomatic/ advanced disease. The study was not conclusive with regard to the progression of internal derangement, as although patients can remain at earlier stages, most of the intermediate cases tended to progress. Internal derangement was less common in older patients, but those with late-stage disease tended to be older and have had symptoms for longer. Younger patients (<25 years) were more likely to have intermediate-stage disease.

The cause of internal derangements remains unclear but is attributed to trauma rather than occlusal or muscular factors. These are proposed to be manifestations rather than causes of internal derangements. In this population, stress was not an issue. The conclusion is that internal derangements represent an organic, progressive disorder.

Study Limitations

This retrospective study was mainly descriptive, lacking statistical analysis of the results. The diagnostic criteria used for the analysis of tomography, arthrography, or MRI are not described, nor was the blinding of radiological analysis for clinical or surgical findings or how the radiological findings were standardised. There is inherent bias in the study design in selecting patients who underwent surgery without fully describing the clinical or radiological criteria for performing surgery and comparing these to the larger cohort of patients who did not undergo surgery. Another limitation is that MRI was not available in the early period of the study, and the use of MRI, and similarly the selection of patients for pathological analysis, was not described.

Relevant Studies

Schellhas et al.[1] performed a study of 743 consecutive arthrograms, and 1,052 TMJs were studied by means of an MRI scan. Forty-three joints were studied with both modalities and the results were correlated to surgical findings. They recommended MRI to be the procedure of choice for diagnosis of uncomplicated internal derangements, whereas arthrography should be performed whenever capsular adhesions or perforations are suspected and whenever MRI is inconclusive. Pullinger[2] stated that radiographic condylar concentricity cannot serve as a characteristic of a normal joint because of its high variability. Ireland[3] in 1953 and more recently Farrar[4] described that internal derangement of the TMJ commonly causes symptoms of clicking and locking. The latter described reciprocal clicking where the click during mandibular retrusion does not occur unless it is preceded by the click during opening. Westesson et al.[5] studied morphology, internal derangement, and joint function in 58 randomly selected autopsy specimens of the TMJ. Morphologic alterations were rarely present in joints with superior disc position. Disc deformation was observed in 31% of joints with partially anterior disc position, and in 77% of the joints with completely anteriorly positioned discs. In the last group, irregularities of the articular surface were present in 65%.

Disc position, however, may be quite variable in asymptomatic individuals.[6,7] In the asymptomatic adult, there is a high prevalence of anterior and mediolateral displacement of the disc, suggesting that abnormal disc position alone may not be sufficient to produce signs and symptoms of TMJ dysfunction. Other studies[8] show a high correlation between partial or complete anterior disc displacement as well as deformation of the disc and osteoarthrosis. Progressive cartilage breakdown eventually leads to denudation of the subchondral bone.[9] In some cases, however, resolution depends on the adaptive powers of the joint, namely the ability of the condyle to remodel in response to the altered position of the meniscus. Eventually, bony remodelling may lead to the end stage of osteoarthrosis,[10] with crepitus being the major clinical symptom, while most clinical signs of previous stages tend to subside. Wilkes' findings that stress was not an issue was also found in the study of Lundeen.[11] It appears that if joint physiologic capacity is not exceeded, use or disuse will not have adverse consequences[12] even in patients with bruxism.[13]

Muscular hyperactivity due to emotional stress, as well as long-standing malocclusion, may become important once articular cartilage breakdown has already started though.[9] Studies suggest that changes in biochemistry and pathophysiology of the synovial fluid and articular and synovial surfaces play an important early role in the pathogenesis of many TMJ disorders. Disc displacement symptoms may be a later secondary phenomenon as a result of altered joint physiology and lubrication.[14]

Nitzan and Dolwick[15] in 1991 presented some doubts as to the validity of the natural history of internal derangements as proposed by Wilkes. Clinical and surgical data of 194 operated joints were studied, and no correlation between increasing age and the stages of the process was found. Also, more than 50% of the discs with a closed lock were normally shaped. They stated that a severely restricted mouth opening of 15–25 mm associated with severely impeded protrusive and lateral movements towards the unaffected side is attributed to a complete restriction of condyle–disc translation on the articular eminence, and not only to a nonreducible, displaced disc. Another question mark placed is the reversibility of the locking situation in the intermediate stage. Reversibility cannot be explained if the only cause is an anteriorly displaced, deformed disc that causes obstruction. Arthroscopic treatment of the upper joint compartment appears to be effective in reestablishing normal joint movement in patients with severe closed lock. The success of these treatments is remarkable considering that these approaches—lavage and lysis,[16,17] pressured injection,[18] and arthrocenthesis of the superior joint space—do not change either disc location or shape. The effect can be attributed to treatment of the lack of gliding due to adherence of the disc to the fossa by a reversible effect such as a vacuum, decreased volume of synovial fluid, or high viscosity. This new look at internal derangements is commended by Israel,[14] who suggested that other conditions may account for symptoms or may coexist with internal derangement. Another interesting study was performed by Emshoff and Rudisch.[19] In a study of 163 patients, the authors found a poor correlation between a standardised clinical evaluation of patients with TMJ internal derangement and osteoarthrosis and the findings of a separate MRI evaluation.

The Wilkes classification is widely and regularly used and forms a basis to stage internal derangements. Further research is needed to evaluate if other pathologic mechanisms and findings can supplement this classification. Furthermore, more longitudinal studies are needed to evaluate the optimal clinical and radiological evaluation.

REFERENCES

1. Schellhas KP, Wilkes CH, Omile MR, et al. The diagnosis of temporomandibular joint disease: two-compartment arthrography and MR. Am J Roentgenol. 1988; 151: 341–50.
2. Pullinger AG, Hollender T, Solberg WK, et al. A tomographic study of mandibular condyle position in an asymptomatic population. J Prost Dent. 1985; 53: 706.
3. Ireland VE. The problem of the "clicking jaw". Proc R Soc Med. 1951; 44: 191.

4. Farrar WB, McCarty WL. Inferior joint space arthrography and characteristics of condylar paths in internal derangements of the TMJ. J Prosthet Dent. 1979; 41: 548–55.
5. Westesson P, Bronstein SL, Liedberg J. Internal derangement of the temporomandibular joint: morphologic description with correlation to joint function. Oral Surg Oral Med Oral Pathol. 1985; 59: 323–31.
6. Moore JB. Coronal and sagittal TMJ meniscus position in asymptomatic subjects by MRI. J Oral Maxillofac Surg. 1989; 47: 75–6.
7. Westesson P, Eriksson L, Kurita K. Reliability of negative clinical temporomandibular joint examination: prevalence of disk displacement in asymptomatic temporomandibular joints. Oral Surg Oral Med Oral Pathol. 1989; 68: 551–4.
8. Westesson P, Rohlin M. Internal derangement related to osteoarthrosis in temporomandibular autopsy specimens. Oral Surg Oral Med Oral Pathol. 1984; 57: 17–22.
9. Stegenga B, de Bont LGM, Boering G. Osteoarthrosis as the cause of craniomandibular pain and dysfunction: a unifying concept. J Oral Maxillofac Surg. 1989; 47: 249–256.
10. Ogus H. The mandibular joint: internal rearrangement. Br J Oral Maxillofac Surg. 1987; 25: 218–26.
11. Lundeen TF, Sturdevant JR, George JM. Stress as a factor in muscle and temporomandibular joint pain. J Oral Rehabil. 1987; 14: 445–56.
12. Radin EL. Biomechanical Considerations. Osteoarthritis, Diagnosis and Management. Philadelphia: Saunders, 1984.
13. Møller E. Discussion. In: Klineberg I, Sessle D. (Eds.) Oro-facial pain and neuromuscular dysfunction: mechanisms and clinical correlates: proceedings of the symposium sponsored by the International commission on oral physiology of the International union of physiological sciences, the Neuroscience group of the International association for dental research and the Australian prosthodontic society 5-6 August 1983, Sydney, Australia. Oxford: Pergamon Press, 1985.
14. Israel HA. An alternative explanation for the genesis of closed-lock symptoms in the internal derangement process. J Oral Maxillofac Surg. 1991; 49: 815–816.
15. Nitzan DW, Dolwick MF. An alternative explanation for the genesis of closed-lock symptoms in the internal derangement process. J Oral Maxillofac Surg. 1991; 49: 810–815.
16. Nitzan DW, Dolwick FM, Heft M. Arthroscopic lavage and lysis of the temporomandibular joint. A change in perspective. J Oral Maxillofac Surg. 1990; 48: 798.
17. Sanders B. Arthroscopic surgery of the temporomandibular joint. Treatment of internal derangement with persistent closed lock. Oral Surg. 1986; 62: 361.
18. Murakami KI, Iizuka T, Matsuki M, et al. Recapturing the persistent anteriorly displaced disk by mandibular manipulation after pumping and hydraulic pressure to the upper joint cavity of the temporomandibular joint. J Craniomandibular Pract. 1987; 5: 17.
19. Emshoff R, Rudisch A. Clinical versus magnetic resonance imaging diagnosis of temporomandibular joint internal derangement and osteoarthrosis. Oral Surg Oral Med Oral Pathol Oral Radiol Endod. 2001; 91: 50–5.

CHAPTER **41**

Symptoms of Temporomandibular Joint Osteoarthrosis and Internal Derangement 30 Years after Non-Surgical Treatment

De Leeuw R, Boering G, Stegenga B, De Bont LGM. Cranio. 1995; 13: 81–8.

Reviewed by Andrew Sidebottom

Research Question/Objective

The existing assumption was that temporomandibular joint osteoarthrosis (TMJ OA) and internal derangement (ID) were progressive disorders whereby a click progresses to locking, restriction, and ultimately disc or retrodiscal tear and degenerative joint disease. The aim of the study was to investigate a group of patients managed nonoperatively, with a diagnosis of TMJ OA or ID at 30 years post-diagnosis, to determine whether, or how, their disease had progressed.

Study Design

The records of 400 patients managed over 30 years ago for craniomandibular pain or dysfunction were screened. Patients were included if their current age was between 50 and 70 years, there was no other diagnosed craniomandibular disorder, and they were able to attend for a consultation. Their records were reviewed by two observers independently to establish eligibility and confirm a diagnosis of reducible (RDD) or permanent disc displacement (PDD).

From the historic patient records, the presence or absence of TMJ or muscle symptoms, joint noises, and parafunction were recorded.

A questionnaire-based assessment was used at a recall visit to establish past treatment, treatment in the interim, and interference of the disorder with masticatory function at present.

A control group consisted of volunteers who had not had and did not currently have TMJ symptoms.

Sample Size

A total of 99 patients treated between 1958 and 1962 were found to be eligible and reviewed at least 30 years later.

The control group consisted of 35 age and sex matched subjects from a current asymptomatic group.

Study Limitations

Despite a large initial sample size, the exclusion criteria led to 75% of the group not being included.

The initial diagnosis was based on a retrospective review of case notes 30 years old by two independent observers agreeing a diagnosis of DD.

The diagnostic criteria have now been superseded by better criteria and therefore it is not absolutely clear whether some symptoms were related to "joint disease" and not myofascial pain. Radiographic examination was limited to plain transcranial radiographs showing "structural changes." Numerous "nonsurgical" managements were utilised, including steroid injections which potentially give a "chemical synovectomy."

Results

The treatment modalities most frequently used in the past were reassurance, exercises, superficial heat, and intra-articular injections. These were used variably in 65% of patients. Occlusal adjustment and oral rehabilitation were used selectively but never undertaken in isolation.

There were no significant differences found in treatment, or symptom duration, between the RDD and PDD groups, with 63% reporting symptom improvement within 3 months, a further 21% between 3 and 6 months, and 6% requiring more than 12 months treatment. At 30 years post treatment, no patients reported significant symptoms, with 90% able to chew undisturbed.

Both the PDD and RDD groups reported some difficulty in opening wide, with the PDD reporting this significantly more frequently, although significantly less than at initial presentation.

In 75% of the RDD group, clicking ceased, with 13% going on to report crepitus compared with 15% reducing to 7% with crepitus in the PDD group. This was felt to be due to adaptation of the joint with remodelling.

Fourteen percent of patients included in the study reported the development of symptoms on the contralateral side during the follow-up period, but none had sought treatment for this.

Masticatory muscle fatigue was more commonly noted in the RDD group than either the PDD or controls. Parafunctional habits were noted more commonly in the RDD and control groups than the PDD group.

Only 3% of the group had requested further treatment for TMJ problems in the intervening years.

There were generally more complaints of musculoskeletal symptoms over the 30-year period, including joint noises, pain, and stiffness, but no difference between the patient and control groups.

Limitations of Study

There were insufficient cases to allow detailed subgroup analysis, and therefore no indication of which patients might progress or would benefit from surgical intervention. The same research group highlighted that early arthrocentesis benefits patients in the long term [1,2] and is more cost-effective.

Diagnostic capabilities were limited to plain radiographs which could not differentiate between osteoarthrosis and remodelling. Even in the current age, CT and MRI cannot differentiate these[3,4] and arthroscopy is more accurate.[4,5]

Key Findings

The key message from this paper is that the majority of patients with disc displacement do not progress to significant degenerative joint disease. Symptoms will mostly improve with simple conservative measures and very few require surgical intervention. In both the patient and control groups, 90% were happy with their joint function, despite some having pain or restriction of wide opening. Disc position does not seem to predict progression to degenerative changes, as indicated by the presence of crepitus.

In the vast majority of cases, clicking will settle over time, and in most cases this will not be replaced by crepitus. Most patients will have minor ongoing issues which are manageable. The presence of crepitus and minor symptoms do not necessarily imply degenerative changes which require intervention.

In light of this paper, then, a much more conservative approach to management of disc displacement is suggested, whereas a more active approach to management of limited joint function after 3–6 months of failed conservative treatment can be justified.

The subsequent introduction of minimally invasive treatments allows easier and more predictable diagnosis and therapeutic benefits,[6,7] but conservative management does not harm the patient and in the long term will benefit the majority.

Current TMJ surgeons are therefore still seeking a method for determining which patients will benefit from early intervention with minimally invasive techniques and which will obtain the same outcome with conservative measures alone.

REFERENCES

1. Vos LM, Huddleston-Slater JJ, Stegenga B. Arthrocentesis as initial treatment for temporomandibular joint arthropathy: a randomized controlled trial. J Craniomaxillofac Surg. 2014; 42: 134–9.
2. Vos LM, Stegenga B, Stant AD, Quik EH, Huddleston-Slater JJ. Cost effectiveness of arthrocentesis compared to conservative therapy for arthralgia of the temporomandibular joint: a randomized controlled trial. J Oral Facial Pain Headache. 2018; 32: 198–207.
3. Shen P, Huo L, Zhang SY, et al. Magnetic resonance imaging applied to the diagnosis of perforation of the temporomandibular joint. J Craniomaxillofac Surg. 2014; 42: 874–8.
4. Yura S, Harada S, Kobayashi K. Diagnostic accuracy on magnetic resonance imaging for the diagnosis of osteoarthritis of the temporomandibular joint. J Clin Diagn Res. 2015; 9: 95–7.
5. Tzanidakis K, Sidebottom AJ. How accurate is arthroscopy of the temporomandibular joint? A comparison of findings in patients who had open operations after arthroscopic management failed. Br J Oral Maxillofac Surg. 2013; 51: 968–70.
6. Ahmed N, Sidebottom A, O'Connor M, Kerr H-L. Prospective outcome assessment of the therapeutic benefits of arthroscopy and arthrocentesis of the temporomandibular joint. Br J Oral Maxillofac Surg. 2012; 50: 745–8.
7. Weedon S, Ahmed N, Sidebottom AJ. Prospective assessment of outcomes following disposable arthroscopy of the TMJ. Br J Oral Maxillofac Surg. 2013; 51: 625–9.

CHAPTER 42

Temporomandibular Joint Arthrocentesis: A Simplified Treatment for Severe, Limited Mouth Opening

Nitzan DW, Dolwick MF, Martinez GA. J Oral Maxillofac Surg. 1991; 49: 1163–7.

Reviewed by Jason Green

Research Question/Objective

The study was designed to investigate the effect of lavage (upper space arthrocentesis) alone in the management of chronic closed lock.

Study Design

A prospective, nonrandomised, uncontrolled study involving case series in two centres in Israel and Florida, USA. Ten patients were treated in one centre and seven in the other.

Sample Size

A total of 17 patients were included in the study: 14 females and 3 males.

Follow-up

Patients were followed up for between 4 and 14 months.

Inclusion/Exclusion Criteria

All patients included in the study had failed to respond to conservative measures of medication, bite splint therapy, physiotherapy, and joint manipulation. All patients had a maximum mouth opening (MMO) of less than 30 mm. Patients who were known to have evidence of fibrous adhesions were excluded.

Intervention or Treatment Received

Prior to treatment, the MMO and lateral excursions were measured (mm) and patients were asked to record pain on a visual analogue score (VAS I 0–15 mm) together with functional disturbance (VAS II 0-15 mm). At follow-up, the same parameters were measured, and a third scale used (VAS III –7 to +7) for self-evaluation of improvement or deterioration.

Patients in the study underwent two needle arthrocentesis of the TMJ under local anaesthetic. The joint was irrigated with 200 ml of Ringer's lactate solution over a 15–20 minute period. During the procedure the patient was asked to make repeated attempts to open the mouth to establish normal mouth opening. Following arthrocentesis, steroid was injected into the joint (6 mg betamethasone). All patients received postoperative analgesia (naproxen sodium 275 mg tds), and diazepam (2.5–5 mg) nocte and were instructed to wear their bite splint at night. Physiotherapy was commenced immediately postsurgery, although exactly what techniques were used was not reported.

Results

The results found that upper space arthrocentesis significantly improved mouth opening ($P < 0.001$), which increased from a range of 12–30 mm (mean, 24.1 ± 5.6 mm) to 35–50 mm (mean 42.7 ± 4 mm). Lateral excursions also improved from 2–6 mm (mean 3.75 ± 2.9) to 8–13 mm (mean 10.5 ± 1.0 mm). Only four patients experienced clicking post treatment compared to twelve at the start of the study. Patients also reported a significant reduction ($P < 0.001$) in pain scores after treatment, from a mean rating of 8.75 ± 2.82 mm (range 3 to 13 mm) to 2.31 ± 2.55 mm (range 0 to 11 mm) when recorded using VAS. Finally, patients reported a significant reduction in functional disturbance ($P < 0.001$) from 10.24 ± 1.72 (range 8–13 mm) down to 2.16 ± 3 mm (range 0.9–11 mm). In terms of overall success, patient reported a 91% improvement in symptoms (self-assessment score 6.4 ± 0.9).

Similar outcomes (in terms of MMO, pain reduction, and improved jaw function) were found in patients from both centres.

Study Limitations

Although a prospective two-centre study, the numbers of subjects included in the study was small. Follow-up times were variable between patients and centres and some of the data recorded was different between the two centres. The type of bite splint and physiotherapy regime is not specified in the study, although the same physiotherapy regime was used pre- and post-treatment.

Relevant Studies

Historically, before the advent of minimal access surgery, the treatment of acute closed lock would consist of open joint surgery. The advent of arthroscopic surgery[1] led to a more conservative approach to the management of internal derangement, reducing the morbidity and potential long-term sequelae of open joint surgery.[2]

Arthrocentesis has less potential risks than arthroscopic surgery,[3,4] but until this study was performed, it was not clear that similar results could be obtained using lavage alone. Subsequent studies[5–8] have shown that arthocentesis can reduce pain from internal derangement and can offer improvements in maximal mouth opening. Arthrocentesis does not require specialist training in arthroscopic techniques, rendering it widely available to all maxillofacial surgeons who treat TMJ patients but who lack the training or confidence to undertake TMJ arthroscopy.[9] A Cochrane review[10] has shown that outcomes from both techniques are comparable but highlight the lack of quality evidence in this area.

Minimally invasive treatment for TMJ dysfunction also has the benefit that it can be repeated with continued improved benefits[11] without causing long-term damage to the joint. It can also be carried out under local or general anaesthetic; however, there are some suggestions that better results may be achieved under general anaesthetic.[12] Arthrocentesis also offers a cost-effective treatment for TMJ internal derangement, as there is no requirement for specialist equipment.[13]

The long-term effectiveness of arthrocentesis has been reported in several studies. Other studies report 79 to 95% success rates in patients followed for up to three years following surgery.[14–16]

REFERENCES

1. Ohnishi M. Arthroscopy of the temporomandibular joint. J Stomatol Soc Japan. 1975; 42: 207–12.
2. Murakami K, Ito K. Arthroscopy of the temporomandibular joint. In M Watanabe (Ed.): Arthroscopy of Small Joints. Tokyo: Igaku Shoin, 1985.
3. Masashi T, Toshirou K, Seto K, et al. Complications of temporomandibular joint arthroscopy: a retrospective analysis of 301 lysis and lavage procedures performed using the triangulation technique. J Oral Maxillofac Surg. 2000; 58: 500–5.
4. Vaira LA, Raho MT, Soma D, et al. Complications and post-operative sequelae of temporomandibular joint arthrocentesis. Cranio. 2018; 36: 264–7.
5. Ness GM. Temporomandibular joint arthrocentesis for acute or chronic closed lock. J Oral Maxillofac Surg. 1996; 54: 112–20.
6. Sembronio S, Albiero AM, Toro C, Robiony M, Politi M. Is there a role for arthrocentesis in recapturing the displaced disc in patients with closed lock of the temporomandibular joint? Oral Surg Oral Med Oral Pathol Oral Radiol Endod. 2008; 105: 274–80.
7. Chandrashekhar VK, Kenchappa U, Chinnannavar SN, Singh S. Arthrocentesis a minimally invasive method for TMJ disc disorders—A prospective study. J Clin Diagn Res. 2015; 9: 59–62
8. Malik AH, Shah AA. Efficacy of temporomandibular joint arthrocentesis on mouth opening and pain in the treatment of internal derangement of TMJ-A—a clinical study. J Oral Maxillofac Surg. 2014; 13: 244–8.
9. Elledge R, Speculand B, Green J, Attard A. Training in surgery of the temporomandibular joint: perceptions of trainees in oral and maxillofacial surgery in the United Kingdom. Br J Oral Maxillofac Surg. 2016; 54: 941–5.
10. Rigon M, Pereira LM, Bortoluzzi MC, et al. Arthroscopy for temporomandibular disorders. Cochrane Database Syst Rev. 2011; 5: CD006385.

11. Kütük N, Baş B, Kazan D, Yüceer E. Is repeated arthrocentesis beneficial in the treatment of temporomandibular disorders: a retrospective study. J Oral Maxillofac Surg. 2019; 77: 1359–64.

12. Tuz HH, Baslarli O, Adiloglu S, Gokturk T, Meral SE. Comparison of local and general anaesthesia for arthrocentesis of the temporomandibular joint. Br J Oral Maxillofac Surg. 2016; 54: 946–9.

13. Vos LM, Stegenga B, Stant AD, Quik EH, Huddleston Slater JJ. Cost effectiveness of arthrocentesis compared to conservative therapy for arthralgia of the temporomandibular joint: a randomized controlled trial. J Oral Facial Pain Headache. 2018; 32: 198–207.

14. Nitzen DW, Samson B, Better H. Long-term outcome of arthrocentesis for severe closed lock of the temporomandibular joint. J Oral Maxillofac Surg. 1997; 55: 151–8.

15. Hosaka H, Murakami K, Goto K, et al. Outcome of arthrocentesis for temporomandibular joint with closed lock at 3 years follow-up. Oral Surg Oral Med Oral Pathol. 1996; 82: 501–4.

16. Carvajal WA, Laskin DM. Long-term evaluation of arthrocentesis for the treatment of internal derangements of the temporomandibular joint. J Oral Maxillofac Surg. 2000; 58: 852–5.

CHAPTER 43

Arthroscopic Surgery of the Temporomandibular Joint Surgery: Treatment of Internal Derangement with Persistent Closed Lock

Sanders B. Oral Surg Oral Med Oral Pathol. 1986; 62: 361–72.

Reviewed by Florencio Monje

Research Question/Objective

Open temporomandibular joint (TMJ) arthroplasty is recommended for the treatment of internal derangement with closed lock, when nonsurgical therapy has failed. The purpose of this article was to present an alternative approach to the surgical correction of internal derangement of the TMJ with closed lock. This approach includes arthroscopic inspection of the superior compartment and lysis (resection, ablation) of adhesions that form between the disc and the fossa with disc displacement.

Study Design

A retrospective nonrandomised study design, without controls, with only narrative results describing the technique of lysis and lavage after diagnostic TMJ arthroscopic assessment.

Sample Size

A total of 40 arthroscopic procedures in 25 patients. Of these, 15 patients had bilateral and 10 unilateral procedures.

There were 24 female patients and 1 male patient. The age range was 11 years to 51 years, with a mean age of 30 years.

Follow-up

Follow-up ranged from 7–10 months.

Inclusion/Exclusion Criteria

The clinical diagnoses were either internal derangement with persistent closed lock or arthrosis, where symptoms had been present for between 1 and 10 years. All but four patients had preoperative arthrograms.

Intervention or Treatment Received

The arthroscope used was 1.9 mm diameter and the joint puncture technique is very well anatomically explained. The first step was diagnostic examination of the TMJ. Different areas to be examined were described and findings such as fibrillations, adhesions, masses of synovial tissues, synovitis, changes in the vascularity, or perforations documented. The surgical technique consisted of an "arthroscopic sweep" of the superior compartment with a blunt trocar, which lyses (resects) the superior compartment adhesions. The superior compartment was thoroughly lavaged by irrigation and suction. A small amount of steroid solution was placed in the superior compartment when the tissues appeared inflamed.

Results

The cases and outcomes are described in Table 43.1. The initial phase of each of the 40 arthroscopies was diagnostic. Fourteen procedures were followed by arthrotomy with meniscectomy, arthroplasty, and insertion of a silicone fossa implant. Twenty-six procedures were therapeutic. Arthroscopic surgery was employed in 21 joints to eliminate persistent closed lock symptoms by lysing superior-compartment adhesions. Arthroscopy was therapeutic in five arthritic joints as well, with lysis of adhesions, lavage, steroid placement, synovectomy, and partial meniscectomy.

The initial postoperative course of patients who underwent therapeutic arthroscopy was good or excellent. All patients who had symptoms of closed lock were essentially asymptomatic, with little preauricular pain and a good range of mouth opening. The arthrosis cases were also significantly improved. Of the 40 arthroscopies, only one complication occurred: a severe postoperative middle ear infection developed in a patient who underwent a unilateral arthroscopy, resulting in hearing impairment.

Study Limitations

This study lacked the essential characteristics of high-quality clinical research such as randomisation or control groups; however, Sanders was the first to report on the symptomatic improvements possible with diagnostic arthroscopy together with lysis and lavage and was the starting point to other more sophisticated techniques.

Relevant Studies

Diagnostic TMJ arthroscopy had previously been reported by Onishi, and several other authors had at this point also described the technique.[1-4] Murakami et al.[2,5] reported successful therapeutic arthroscopic treatment in patients with TMJ closed lock where forcible insertion of a blunt arthroscopic trocar between the fossa and the disc, with a "sweeping" action of the trocar, resulted in ablation of surface adhesions. The disc was then able to mobilise,

Table 43.1 Demographic Characteristics, Type of Treatment and Follow-Up of the Patients

No.	Patient's Age (yr)	Patient's Sex	TMJ	Duration of Symptoms	Clinical Diagnosis	Radiographic Findings	Arthroscopic Examination	Arthroscopic Surgery	Arthrotomy (arthroplasty, meniscectomy, etc.)	Postop. (mo.)	Follow-up Complications
1	30	F	R	5 yr 6 mo	DJD	DJD, NRAD	AES	No	Yes	10	E
2	30	F	L	2 yr	CL	NRAD	AS	Yes	No	10	E
3	47	F	L	5 yr	DJD	DJD	EASP	No	Yes	10	E
4	47	F	R	1 yr	DJD	DJD	EAS	Yes	No	10	E
5	18	F	R	1 yr	CL	NRAD	AS	Yes	No	10	E
6	18	F	L	1 yr	CL	NRAD	AS	Yes	No	10	E
7	39	F	L	6 yr	DJD	DJD	APE	No	Yes	10	E
8	49	F	R	1 yr 6 mo	CL	NRAD	AS	Yes	No	9	E
9	49	F	L	1 yr 6 mo	DJD	DJD	AS	No	Yes	9	F
10	28	F	R	8 yr	DJD	DJD	ASE	Yes	No	9	G
11	28	F	L	8 yr	DJD	DJD	ASE	No	Yes	9	F
12	20	F	R	1 yr 6 mo	CL	NRAD	AS	Yes	No	9	E
13	20	F	L	1 yr 6 mo	CL	NRAD	AS	Yes	No	9	E
14	30	F	R	1 yr	CL	NRAD	AS	Yes	No	9	E
15	30	F	L	1 yr	CL	NRAD	AS	Yes	No	9	E
16	51	F	R	3 yr	DJD	DJD	ASE	Yes	No	8	E
17	51	F	L	3 yr	DJD	DJD	ASE	No	Yes	8	G
18	19	F	L	2 yr	CL	NRAD	AS	Yes	No	8	E
19	25	F	R	10 yr	DJD	DJD	ASE	No	Yes	8	G
20	25	F	L	10 yr	DJD	DJD	ASE	Yes	Yes	8	G
21	24	F	R	2 yr 6 mo	DJD	DJD	ASE	No	Yes	8	G
22	24	F	L	2 yr	DJD	DJD	ASE	No	Yes	8	G
23	23	F	L	10 yr	CL	NRAD	AS	No	No	8	E
24	11	F	L	Yr 6 mo	CL	NRAD	AS	Yes	No	8	E

(Continued)

Table 43.1 (Continued)

No.	Patient's Age (yr)	Patient's Sex	TMJ	Duration of Symptoms	Clinical Diagnosis	Radiographic Findings	Arthroscopic Examination	Arthroscopic Surgery	Arthrotomy (arthroplasty, meniscectomy, etc.)	Postop. (mo.)	Follow-up	Complications
25	46	F	L	Yr 6 mo	CL	NRAD	AS	Yes	No	8	G	
26	35	M	R	2 yr	CL	NRAD	AS	Yes	No	8	UNK	Severe ear infection, resultant hearing defect
27	37	F	R	3 mo	CL	NRAD	AS	Yes	No	8	E	
28	19	F	R	3 mo	CL	NRAD	AS	Yes	No	8	E	
29	19	F	L	3 mo	CL	NRAD	AS	Yes	No	8	E	
30	25	F	L	1 yr	DJD	DJD	ASE	No	Yes	7	E	
31	30	F	L	10 yr	DJD	DJD	ASE	No	Yes	7	G	
32	32	F	R	2 yr	CL	NRAD	AS	Yes	No	7	E	
33	32	F	L	2 yr	CL	NRAD	AS	Yes	No	7	E	
34	28	F	R	1 yr	CL	NRAD	AS	Yes	No	7	E	
35	28	F	L	1 yr	CL	NRAD	AS	Yes	No	7	E	
36	28	F	R	6 mo	DJD	DJD	ASE	No	Yes	7	G	
37	28	F	L	6 mo	DJD	DJD	ASE	No	Yes	7	G	
38	27	F	R	11 mo	CL, DJD	DJD	ASEP	Yes	No	7	E	
39	27	F	L	11 mo	CL, DJD	DJD	ASE	Yes	No	7	E	
40	25	F	L	1 mo	CL	NRAD	AS	Yes	No	7	E	

DJD = Degenerative joint disease
CL = Closed lock (persistent)
E (follow-up) = Excellent
G = Good
UNK = Unknown, lost to follow-up
E = Eburnation
P = Perforated disc
NRAD = Non-reducing anteriorly displaced disc
A = Adhesions
S = Synovitis
P = Perforated disc

and the closed lock was eliminated. The procedure presented in this article is a variation of Murakami's technique.

Sanders was the first author to report on the beneficial effects of arthroscopy of the TMJ in specific conditions. It was presented as a minimally invasive and effective surgical technique for cases of acute or chronic closed lock of the TMJ. The technique, as mentioned above, involved establishing two approaches or entries, a diagnostic examination of the upper compartment, the removal of the adhesions with a blunt trocar, lavage, and injection of a corticoid solution. A later article by Sanders and Buoncristiani[6] described their 2-year clinical experience of using this technique. Some 82% of the patients presented excellent results (maximum mouth opening of 40 mm or more with little or no joint pain), 14% had good results, and only 4% had poor results.

Indresano[7] analysed the results of 64 patients (100 arthroscopic operations) after a follow-up of 9 to 30 months, considering three parameters: mouth opening, reduction of postoperative pain according to the VAS (visual analogue scale), and the need for some type of subsequent treatment. Improvement was noted in 73% of the patients, with the best results in cases of acute or chronic locking (83% with improvement). Less pain was appreciated by 70% of the patients.

Montgomery[8] studied the lysis and lavage in 19 patients with a follow-up of 6 to 12 months, showing that 90% of the patients improved, despite 50% having some residual pain. The postoperative treatment was variable and therefore it was not possible to determine to what degree the results were due to the joint lysis and lavage.

Moses et al.[9] reviewed 152 joints with disc displacement without reduction in which lysis was laterally applied to adhesions with the use of blunt and pointed trocars. These authors advise making several anterior-posterior movements with the cannula and a blunt trocar in order not only to break the adhesions but also to eliminate the herniation of the lateral capsule that accompanies these types of cases. Some 92% of the patients showed pain reduction and 78% had a maximum mouth opening of 40 mm. This classical paper analysed pre- and postoperative MRI, demonstrating that 92% of the patients had persistent, non-reducing anteriorly displaced discs, although 80% of patients experienced marked improvement in disc mobility.

In the same year, Moses and Poker[10] reported the results of 237 patients with an average follow-up period of 19 months. This time, 92% of the patients presented reduced pain and increased mouth opening. The presence of perforation in the bilaminar zone and degenerative joint disease did not appear to alter the results; however, the presence of condylar osteophytes was associated with a poorer prognosis.

Perrot et al.[11] in a prospective study of 76 joints treated with lysis and lavage plus intra-articular corticoid injection, confirmed decreased pain, and increased joint mobility.

In 1991, Clark et al.[12] found pain reduction (using VAS) in 57% of patients, while 83% had a mouth opening of 30 to 43 mm in patients with disc displacement without reduction. These authors concluded that disc position was of minor importance in the symptoms of the patient, as lysis and lavage did not alter the position of the disc.

Davis et al.[13] used lysis and lavage of adhesions, anterior release and the elimination of irregularities with a motorised element where necessary and reported the maximum mouth opening improved from 28.9 mm to 37.8 mm in bilateral cases.

Moore[14] noted that in 63 patients with 4-year follow-up that the pathology that most improved after this therapy was joint locking. Mosby[15] published a study of 150 joints with non-reducible disc displacement, degenerative joint disease, or fibrous ankylosis. Of these, 93% showed a reduction in pain and 90% were capable of chewing when placed on a normal diet during the postoperative period.

Arthroscopic surgery of the TMJ has become a common procedure, with a great variety of surgical techniques and instruments described. Disc-repositioning techniques, capsular release, synovial coagulation, chondroplasty, discoplasty, and fibrous debridement have all been incorporated in arthroscopic procedures, using manual instruments, rotary mechanical shavers, monopolar or bipolar electrocautery, and lasers.

All of these aim to improve the mobility of the intra-articular disc, and consequently the joint, resulting in improvement in joint pain and mouth opening.

Arthroscopic lysis and lavage has been shown to be quite reliable in achieving these goals in patient with acute and chronic closed lock, particularly before significant degenerative changes such as osteophytes have developed. ,

There is at present relatively little evidence to support one technique over another.

REFERENCES

1. Ohnishi M. Arthroscopy of the temporomandibular joint. J Stomatol Soc Japan. 1975; 42: 207–13.
2. Murakami K, Ito K. Arthroscopy of the temporomandibular joint third report: clinical experiences. Arthroscopy. 1984; 9: 49–59.

3. Hellsing G, Homlund A, Nordenram A, Wredmark T. Arthroscopy of the temporomandibular joint: examination of two patients with suspected disc derangement. Int J Oral Surg. 1984; 13: 69–74.
4. Burke RH. Temporomandibuylar joint diagnosis: arthroscopy. J Craniomandibular Pract. 1985; 3: 233–6.
5. Murakami K, Matsuki M, Iziuka T, Ono T, Hoshino T. Arthroscopic differential diagnoses and treatments of the locking symptoms of the TMJ and their regional anatomical interpretations. Congress of European Association for Maxillofacial Surgery in Paris, 1984, Abstr 89.
6. Sanders B, Buoncristiani R. Diagnostic and surgical arthroscopy of the temporomandibular joint: clinical experience with 137 procedures over a 2-year period. J Craniomandib Disord. 1987; 1: 202–13.
7. Indresano T. Arthroscopic surgery of the temporomandibular jont. J Oral Maxillofac Surg. 1989; 47: 439–41.
8. Montgomery M, Van Sickels J, Harm S. Arthroscopic TMJ surgery. Effects on signs, symptoms and disc position. J Oral Maxillofac Surg. 1989; 47: 1263–71.
9. Moses JJ, Sartoris D, Glass R. The effects of arthroscopic lysis and lavage of the superior joint space on TMJ disc position and mobility. J Oral Maxillofac Surg. 1989; 47: 674–8.
10. Moses JJ, Poker ID. TMJ arthroscopy: an analysis of 237 patients. J Oral Maxillofac Surg. 1989; 47: 790–4.
11. Perrott DH, Alborzi A, Kaban LB. A prospective evaluation of the effectiveness of temporomandibular joint arthroscopy. J Oral Maxillofac Surg. 1990; 48: 1029–32.
12. Clark GT, Moody DG, Sanders B. Arthroscopic treatment of temporomandibular joint locking resulting from disc derangement: two year result. J Oral Maxillofac Surg. 1991; 49: 157–64.
13. Davis EL, Kaminishi RM, Marshall MW. Arthroscopic surgery for treatment of closed lock. J Oral Maxillofac Surg. 1991; 49: 704.
14. Moore LJ. Arthroscopic surgery for the tretament of restrictive temporomandibular joint disease. A prospective longitudinal study. In Clark G, Sanders B, Bertolami C (Eds.): Advances in Diagnostic and Surgical Arthroscopy of the Temporomandibular Joint. Philadelphia: WB Saunders Company, 1993.
15. Mosby EL. Efficacy of temporomandibular joint arthroscopy: a retrospective study. J Oral Maxillofac Surg. 1993; 51: 17–21.

CHAPTER 44

Twenty-Year Follow-Up Study on Patient-Fitted Temporomandibular Joint Prosthesis: The Techmedia/ TMJ Concepts Device

Wolford LM, Mercuri LG, Schneiderman ED, Movahed R, Allen W.
J Oral Maxillofac Surg. 2015; 73: 952–60.

Reviewed by Nadeem R Saeed

Research Questions/Objective

To collate long-term subjective and objective data on patients treated for end-stage temporomandibular joint (TMJ) disease with custom produced alloplastic joint replacements. In particular, the study provided information on jaw pain, diet ability, jaw function, quality of life (QoL), and mouth opening before and after surgery. Further aims included the influence of number of previous surgeries on these outcomes and the longevity of the devices and potential reasons for early removal.

Study Design

A prospective cohort study limited to two-experienced TMJ surgeons (Larry Wolford and Louis Mercuri). Standardised pre- and post-surgical (latest available) data collection forms were evaluated with a minimum follow-up period of 19 years. Subjective data compared pre-surgical with longest follow-up values using Likert scales for pain (0, no pain; 10, worst pain imaginable), jaw function (0, normal function; 10, no movement), diet (0, no restriction; 10 liquid only), and quality of life (improved, the same, or worse). Measuring maximal incisal opening with adjustments for anterior open bite and deep vertical overbite assessed objective evaluation.

Sample Size

The first 111 consecutive patients operated by the two surgeons were enrolled in the study and were treated between 1989 and 1993.

Follow-up

Fifty six (50.5%) of 111 patients, fulfilled the inclusion criteria for analysis including 19 years follow-up, 10 patients had died (9%), and 45 could not be included due to incomplete data or loss to follow-up. Comparison of the baseline characteristics of patients completing the study with those lost to follow-up showed no statistical differences, supporting the contention that patients lost to follow-up were missing at random and did not differ from those that completed the study.

Inclusion/Exclusion Criteria

Patents were only included if they exhibited end-stage TMJ disease, surgery was performed by one of the agreed surgeons, they were contactable and could be evaluated and agreed to participate. The only exclusion criterion was loss to follow-up.

Results

Of the final 56 patients, 52 (93%) were female and 4 (7%) male. Forty-three patients (77%) were bilateral cases and 13 (23%) unilateral with a total of 99 joints implanted. Mean age at surgery was 38.6 years (SD 10 years, range 15–59 years). Median follow-up was 21 years (IQR, 20 to 22 years).

Presurgical and longest follow-up data comparison showed statistically significant improvement (P < 0.001) in pain reduction (8, IQR 2 to 3, IQR 6), jaw function improvement (7.5, IQR 3 to 3, IQR4), diet (7, IQR 3 to 3, IQR 4).

Forty-eight patients (85.7%) reported improved QoL, 6 (10.7%) had no change, and 2 (3.6%) worsened.

Objective maximal incisal opening showed statistically significant improvement (25.8 mm, SD 9.8 mm to 36.2 mm, SD 7.8 mm).

The median number of previous surgeries was 3 (IQR 4, range 0–27). Postoperative pain and limitation in mouth opening were correlated to number of previous surgeries. None of the 56 study patients exhibited prosthesis failure.

The improvement rates for patients in this study suggest that experienced surgeons should achieve good to excellent outcomes and longevity for alloplastic TMJ reconstruction in patients when using patient-fitted (custom-made) TMJ replacements of the appropriate biomaterials.

Study Limitations

The greatest potential issue with the study was the high dropout rate (nearly 50%) raising concerns of bias and the potential that the dropout group were either worse pre-surgery or had poorer outcomes yet are not included. The authors fully address this issue and highlight the similar baseline characteristics between the final study group and dropout group. Although not stated as an aim of the study, it is disappointing that the authors made no real comment on the complications suffered by their patient cohort.

Comment

This study provides excellent data supporting the use of patient-fitted TMJ Concepts joint replacements. It also details longevity information, which can be shared with patients and provides further comment on reduced outcomes in multiply operated patients.

While the aims and indications for TMJ reconstruction are well established, there remains a multitude of techniques available. Autogenous reconstruction may offer biological adaptability and compatibility but often with donor site morbidity and unpredictable outcomes.[1] The costochondral graft frequently results in the need for further surgery.[2] The early failure of alloplastic systems was related to poor material choice and design and resulted in the abandonment of such methods for many years.[3]

This study highlights the need for a well-designed joint of suitable materials fitted by experienced surgeons. In such cases alloplastic reconstruction offers reduced further surgery rates than autogenous reconstruction.[4] These results can be extrapolated to the Zimmer Biomet microfixation system, which uses effectively identical materials in a well-designed system. Studies on this system are emerging.[5] It is unclear whether a stock prosthesis with ultimately a poorer fit and potentially poorer primary stability will behave in a similar fashion.[6]

REFERENCES

1. Khadka A, Hu J. Autogenous grafts for condylar reconstruction in treatment of TMJ ankylosis: current concepts and considerations for the future. Int J Oral Maxillofac Surg. 2012; 41: 94–102.
2. Saeed NR, Kent JN. A retrospective study of the costochondral graft in TMJ reconstruction. Int J Oral Maxillofac Surg. 2003; 32: 606–9.
3. Milam SB. Failed implants and multiple operations. Oral Surg. 1997; 83: 156–62
4. Saeed N, Hensher R, Mcleod N, Kent J. Reconstruction of the temporomandibular joint autogenous compared with alloplastic. Br J Oral Maxillofac Surg. 2002; 40: 296–9.
5. Boyo A, Mckay J, Lebovic G, Psutka DJ. Temporomandibular joint total replacement using the Zimmer Biomet Microfixation patient-matched prosthesis results in reduced pain and improved function. Oral Surg Oral Med Oral Pathol Oral Radiol. 2019; 128: 572–80.
6. Sanovich R, Mehta U, Abramowicz S, Widner C, Dolwick MF. Total alloplastic temporomandibular joint reconstruction using Biomet stock prostheses: the university of Florida experience. Int J Oral Maxillofac Surg. 2014; 43: 1091–5.

CHAPTER 45

Fractures of the Edentulous Mandible: The Chalmers J. Lyons Academy Study

Bruce R, Strachan D. J Oral Surg. 1976; 34: 973–9.

Reviewed by Indran Balasundaram and Mike Perry

Research Question/Objective

There is a greater rate of non-union in fractures of the atrophic edentulous mandible. Achieving accurate reduction is difficult and patients are usually elderly, with reduced osteogenesis, blood supply, and atrophic bone, further compounding a favourable outcome. As these fractures are relatively uncommon, surgeons have limited experience and the numbers required for statistical evaluation are not possible by a single surgeon or single unit. The aim of this paper was to evaluate the past experiences of the members of the Chalmers J. Lyons Academy of Oral Surgery, define the problems statistically, and make recommendations on treatment modalities.

Study Design

A retrospective case review was performed via a membership questionnaire, sent to all members of the Chalmers J. Lyons Academy of Oral Surgery relating to each practitioner's experiences. The following variables about the patients were included: age, sex, systemic health before the injury, concomitant injuries, cause of fracture, area of fracture, type of fracture, height of mandibular body at fracture site, position of fragments, time between injury and treatment, method of reduction and fixation, time of fixation, postoperative complications associated with the fracture, systemic complications, results, and follow-up treatment. The results were tabulated and computerised statistics of correlation coefficients and student *t* tests were used.

Sample Size

Information was obtained on 216 patients (the paper does not confirm the response rate).

Inclusion/Exclusion Criteria

Questionnaires were sent to all members. All fracture locations of the edentulous mandible were reported, but the study then focused on fractures of the body and symphysis where the problem of non-union was most common. Therefore, 146 cases were fully evaluated.

Intervention/Treatment Received

66% were treated with some type of open reduction including intra-oral and extra-oral approaches. Wire sutures, wire mesh, Kirschner wires, bone plates, and bone grafts with or without denture or splint wiring were used. Thirty-four percent were treated with the closed technique.

Results

Out of 146 cases studied, 31 (21%) had non union. Twenty-five were treated by open reduction and 6 closed. Older patients had more systemic health problems, thinner mandibles, and more postoperative systemic complications. Patients with more complex fractures were treated later after injury and for longer. Patients with a history of systemic health problems before injury were treated for longer, and patients with bilateral fractures who had open reductions were treated for longer. Patients with a history of systemic health problems had thinner mandibles. Those with previous systemic health problems had more postoperative complications. There was a greater incidence in postoperative complications in those who had open fixation. Open reductions were more commonly performed where there was greater displacement of the fractures. Fractures that were comminuted and compound tended to have greater displacement.

Bilateral fractures were associated with thinner mandibles, especially in older patients. The fractures were also more displaced and had a greater time between injury and treatment. They also had more postoperative complications and non-unions.

The authors concluded that there is a high rate of non-union (20%) in the atrophic fractured edentulous mandible. Ultimately, some sort of stabilisation should be used, but based on their observations they have advised that closed methods should be attempted first if possible, as open reduction is more likely to cause non-union. If the patient can tolerate an operation, bone grafting should be considered. Bone plates should be limited to larger non-atrophic mandibles and wire mesh is preferable if stability is to be gained by a metal appliance. Intramedullary pins do not seem to offer any advantage.

Study Limitations

This paper used a retrospective questionnaire to collect data, but the authors did not state the overall response rate. They did not clarify the demographic of the respondents, for example, their level of expertise. Statistical analysis was performed on their data and conclusions were made from these rather than a clear research question to start with. The authors did not state how the variables were measured. For example, with mandible height, was this measured clinically or from a radiograph? How was this standardised and how was it measured? How was the health status of the patients measured? This is not clear, as is the case for many of the other variables looked at. The authors discuss how postoperative complications were more common in fractures treated openly, but they did not state what these complications were. They concluded that closed methods should be attempted first, as the open surgery was more likely to cause non-union. However, they also stated that less favourable fractures that were comminuted with greater displacement were more likely to be treated openly confounding this conclusion.

Relevant Studies

Knowledge of osteosynthesis and fracture fixation principles with load sharing and load bearing plates has greatly increased since the 1980s. This paper is therefore outdated. Although, it should be recognised it was one of the earliest attempts to provide an experience-based protocol for the management of these difficult patients.

Luhr published a case series in 1996 which classified the degree of atrophy in fractures of the atrophic edentulous mandible.[1] Class 1 atrophy is where the height of the mandible at the fracture site is 16–20 mm. Class 2 is 11–15 mm and class 3 is less than or equal to 10 mm. Eighty-four fractured edentulous mandibles were treated with compression plating (open approach). In six cases bone grafting was used due to a partial bone defect at the fracture site. No postoperative intermaxillary fixation was used. In 81/84 (96.5%) solid bony union was achieved. There were three major complications, two non-unions (both in patients with class 3 mandibular atrophy), and one case of osteomyelitis. Minor infections with no interference with fracture healing were observed in six cases (7%). The authors concluded that for fractures in mandibles with class 3 atrophy periosteal degloving should be avoided and supra-periosteal placement of plates is recommended. They also state that compression osteosynthesis is a successful method.

More recently, Gerbino et al. published a case series of 55 patients with 68 fractures (23 were bilateral) from three Italian trauma centres.[2] Inclusion criteria included atropic edentulous mandible fracture less than 20 mm in height. All patients were treated by open reduction and internal fixation using 2.0 mm or 2.4 mm large profile locking bone plates. No bone grafts were used. All patients achieved complete fracture healing, although reduction was deemed poor in 6/68 fracture sites. The authors concluded that external open reduction and internal fixation is a reliable and predictable treatment and that bone grafting should only be considered if there is bone loss.

Batbayer et al. devised a treatment protocol for fractures of the edentulous mandibles in 2018[3] similar to the above treatment protocols, but they have specified those fractures less than 10 mm in height should be treated with a load-bearing plate with three locking screws on either side of the fracture and a bone graft. Those greater than10 mm should only have a bone graft if there is a continuity defect. In their series of 36 patients with 61 fractures, 53 fractures were treated according to the protocol and 8 were not. Of the 53 following the protocol, 4 had complications (7.5%). Of the 8 not following the protocol, 4 had complications (50%).

Nasser et al. performed a Cochrane review in 2007 on the management of the fractured edentulous atrophic mandible.[4] They did not find any randomised controlled trials and concluded that there was inadequate evidence for the effectiveness of a single approach either open or closed. Until high-level evidence is available, treatment decisions should continue to be based on a clinician's prior experience.

The paper discussed in this chapter has been superseded by a better understanding of fracture healing and osteosynthesis using titanium plates, which can be load bearing or sharing. Most surgeons would agree that if a patient agrees to surgery, an open approach should be used. The question to consider today is whether the open approach should be extra-oral to minimise periosteal stripping rather than an intra-oral approach and when and where bone grafts should be used.

REFERENCES

1. Luhr HG, Reidick T, Merten HA. Results of treatment of fractures of the atrophic edentulous mandible by compression plating: a retrospective evaluation of 84 consecutive cases. J Oral Maxillofac Surg. 1996; 54: 250–4; discussion 254–5.
2. Gerbino G, Cocis S, Roccia F, et al. Management of atrophic mandibular fractures: an Italian multicentric retrospective study. J Craniomaxillofac Surg. 2018; 46: 2176–81.
3. Batbayar EO, Bos RRM, van Minnen B. A treatment protocol for fractures of the edentulous mandible. J Oral Maxillofac Surg. 2018; 76: 2151–60.
4. Nasser M, Fedorowicz Z, Ebadifar A. Management of the fractured edentulous atrophic mandible. Cochrane Database Syst Rev. 2007; 24: CD006087.

CHAPTER 46

Open versus Closed Treatment of Fractures of the Mandibular Condylar Process: A Prospective Randomised Multi-Centre Study

Eckelt U, Schneider M, Erasmus F, et al.
J Craniomaxillofac Surg. 2006; 34: 306–14.

Reviewed by Henry Leonhardt and Adrian Franke

Research Question/Objective

Selecting between open and closed treatment of mandibular condyle fractures is still controversial, though many studies have attempted to clarify this problem. Open reduction and internal fixation seem to obtain better results, but one has to consider the difficulties of the surgical approach and the risks of the operation. The aim of the study was to compare both strategies in treatment of moderately displaced condylar fractures and/or fractures with shortening of the mandibular ramus in a prospective and randomised multicentre study.

Study Design

An international prospective and randomised multicentre study assessed the results of open versus closed treatment of moderately displaced condylar fractures. Objective parameters such as radiographic measurements, clinical, functional and subjective parameters such as visual analogue scale for pain, and the Mandibular Function Impairment Questionnaire (MFIQ) index for dysfunction were evaluated.

Sample Size

Seven contributing centres observed 88 patients. Of these, 66 patients with a total of 79 fractures of the mandibular condylar process were included.

Follow-up

Patients were evaluated 6 weeks and 6 months after treatment. At these points, clinical parameters (range of motion: mouth opening, lateral excursion and protrusion, deviation and deflection during mouth opening, malocclusion), subjective parameters (MFIQ and VAS for pain and discomfort, malocclusion), and radiographic results (accuracy of fracture reduction and stability of fixation) were assessed.

Inclusion/Exclusion Criteria

Patients over 18 years of age with uni- or bilateral fractures of the condylar base, the condylar neck, or the condyle itself were included in the study if the displacement of the condylar fragment was between 10 and 45° in frontal or sagittal plane and/or there was shortening of the height of the ascending ramus of 2 mm or more.

Patients were excluded if they had had preexisting skeletal deformations with malocclusions or pathological conditions of the temporomandibular joint. Patients lacking capacity or the ability to consent and fully cooperate were also excluded.

Intervention or Treatment Received

Patients were allocated in two treatment groups: closed treatment and operative treatment. The closed treatment group (n = 30) was usually treated by short-term elastic maxillomandibular immobilisation applied to arch bars for 10 days. This was occasionally prolonged in cases with complications. A phase of functional treatment or physiotherapy and orthodontic appliances followed. Operative treatment implied open reduction and internal fixation of the fracture. In the operative treatment group (n = 36), different surgical approaches (submandibular-, periangular-, retromandibular-, preauricular-, and transoral approaches) and osteosynthesis systems (miniplates, miniscrews, and lag screws) were applied depending on the preference of the operating centre and the height of fracture.

Results

There were no severe complications in either group.

With regard to the radiographic results there was no statistical differences found between the two groups before treatment. After 6 months the ramus height (5.75 mm; range 0–15 mm, SD 4 mm) and degree of angulation (16.8°; range 0–45°, SD 14.6°) within the closed treatment group were unchanged, whereas ramus heights and angulations had significantly improved in the open treatment group.

A significantly better outcome for functional parameters was observed in the open treatment group. Mouth opening and protrusion were superior to the closed treatment group (average interincisal distance 46.5 mm (SD 5.3 mm) versus 40.9 mm (SD 6.7 mm) (p = 0.01), protrusion 7.3 mm (SD 2.0 mm) versus 4.7 mm (SD 25 mm) (p = 0.0005). The amount of laterotrusion in the open treatment group was higher than in the group of closed treatment, but this difference was not statistically significant. In the closed treatment group, 66%

of the patients had a deflection of the mandible during mouth opening (3.1 mm), but only 19% of the patients in the open treatment group (2.6 mm) (p = 0.03).

With regard to malocclusion, there were only 3 subjective (9%) and no objective (0%) malocclusions in the open treatment group after 6 months versus 7 subjective (23%) and 6 objective (20%) malocclusions in the closed treatment group.

The patients with open treatment showed better results concerning pain and discomfort. The evaluation of these subjective parameters assessed by VAS and MFIQ revealed a statistically significant advantage for the open treatment group over the closed treatment group.

Study Limitations

The results of this study showed a clear benefit for the open treatment of condylar neck fractures. The follow-up was only 6 months, but Haug and Assael[1] found that the long-term results of open and closed treatment are similar. Nevertheless, there is consensus that open treatment leads to good functional results more swiftly.

Another limitation is the group sample, which contains uni- and bilateral condylar neck fractures. Closed treatment of bilateral condylar neck fractures with the inclusion criteria of this study will lead to significantly worse results than open treatment because of the lack of support of the healthy side in functional treatment. An additional limitation is the mixture of intra- and extracapsular fractures, i.e., condylar neck and diacapitular fractures of the mandible.

Due to the different approaches in the open treatment, a correction of the disc position and tightening of the articular capsule is possible and could improve functional results compared to the open treatment of condylar neck fractures. In closed treatment, improvement in position of the condylar neck fragment is theoretically possible by the use of a hypomochlion, which is not possible in diacapitular fractures of the mandible because of the traction of the pterygoid muscles on the condylar head fragment. Nowadays there are clearer classifications that can overcome the differentiation of the above-mentioned fractures as suggested by Neff et al.[2]

The results of closed treatment are strongly dependent on the functional treatment after the intermaxillary fixation. A clear therapy standard for maxillomandibular fixation and following functional therapy for the closed treatment of the participating centres may have improved the results of the closed treatment group. In open treatment with perfect reduction of the fracture, results are more comparable despite different fixation techniques.

Relevant Studies

The question of open versus closed treatment of condylar process fractures of the mandible has been discussed over years and many studies suggest benefits for the open treatment of condylar process fractures. Newer literature suggests open treatment,[3,4] but in 2000 Ellis[5] had already published that open treatment was superior to closed treatment regarding occlusal results. However, the follow-up has to be long enough to study the results of closed treatment.

In 2001, Haug and Assael[1] reported the long-term results of open versus closed treatment and found no statistically significant difference between the two groups for functional results, but the closed treatment group was associated with chronic pain. In 2010, Danda et al.[6] found no significant difference in TMJ pain and functional results between both groups. There was, however, a radiographically better anatomic reduction of the condylar process in the open treatment group. Nevertheless, there is a strong consensus in the literature about better functional results of open treatment in bilateral condylar fractures, which was clearly demonstrated in the studies of Newman in 2008 and Singh in 2012.[7,8]

In 2015, a meta-analysis by Berner[9] suggests better functional results and less pain for open treatment but states also clearly, that due to different study protocols and lack of information on classification, follow-up time, and inclusion criteria, comparison of the studies was difficult. In the same year, Chrcanovic[10] found statistically significant effects for functional results favouring open treatment in a meta-analysis. There was a decreased rate of infection in closed treatment and no effects on TMJ-pain.

A review of the literature by Kommers in 2013[11] stated that there was no study dealing with the quality of life after open versus closed treatment to date. Quality of life is the most significant outcome following the treatment of fractures of the mandibular condyle, and some studies, including this one, attempt to consider quality of life by means of subjective assessment of mandibular function and patient related outcome measures, using tools such as the Mandibular Function Impairment Questionnaire, and further studies should include such outcome measures.[12]

REFERENCES

1. Haug RH, Assael LA. Outcomes of open versus closed treatment of mandibular subcondylar fractures. J Oral Maxillofac Surg. 2001; 59: 370–5; discussion 375–6.
2. Neff A, Cornelius CP, Rasse M, Torre DD, Audigé L. The comprehensive AOCMF classification system: condylar process fractures. Craniomaxillofac Trauma Reconstr. 2014; 7: S044–S058.
3. Kotrashetti SM, Lingaraj JB, Khurana V. A comparative study of closed versus open reduction and internal fixation (using retromandibular approach) in the management of subcondylar fracture. Oral Surg Oral Med Oral Pathol Oral Radiol. 2013; 115: e7–e11.

4. Shiju M, Rastogi S, Gupta P, et al. Fractures of the mandibular condyle–Open versus closed–A treatment dilemma. Craniomaxillofac Surg. 2015; 43: 448–51.

5. Ellis E 3rd, Simon P, Throckmorton GS. Occlusal results after open or closed treatment of fractures of the mandibular condylar process. J Oral Maxillofac Surg. 2000; 58: 260–8.

6. Danda AK, Muthusekhar MR, Narayanan V, Baig MF, Siddareddi A. Open versus closed treatment of unilateral subcondylar and condylar neck fractures: a prospective, randomized clinical study. J Oral Maxillofac Surg. 2010; 68: 1238–41.

7. Singh V, Bhagol A, Dhingra R. A comparative clinical evaluation of the outcome of patients treated for bilateral fracture of the mandibular condyles. J Craniomaxillofac Surg. 2012; 40: 464–6.

8. Newman L. A clinical evaluation of the long-term outcome of patients treated for bilateral fracture of the mandibular condyles. Br J Oral Maxillofac Surg. 1998; 36: 176–9.

9. Berner T, Essig H, Schumann P, et al. Closed versus open treatment of mandibular condylar process fractures: a meta-analysis of retrospective and prospective studies. J Craniomaxillofac Surg. 2015; 43: 1404–8.

10. Chrcanovic BR. Surgical versus non-surgical treatment of mandibular condylar fractures: a meta-analysis. Int J Oral Maxillofac Surg. 2015; 44: 158–79.

11. Kommers SC, van den Bergh B, Forouzanfar TJ. Quality of life after open versus closed treatment for mandibular condyle fractures: a review of literature. Craniomaxillofac Surg. 2013; 41: e221–e5.

12. Ologunde R, McLeod NMH. Patient reported outcome measures used in oral and maxillofacial trauma surgery: a literature review. Br J Oral Maxillofac Surg. 2018; 56: 371–9.

CHAPTER 47

The Importance of the Zygomatic Arch in Complex Midfacial Fracture Repair and Correction of Post-Traumatic Orbitozygomatic Deformities

Gruss JS, Wyck LV, Phillips JH, Antonyshyn O. Plast Reconstr Surg. 1990; 85: 878–90.

Reviewed by Harald Essig

Research Question/Objective

In this study, the authors highlighted that the zygomatic arch is a key area for adequate reduction of the outer facial frame in primary midfacial trauma and in secondary reconstruction of post-traumatic deformities. Specific anatomic landmarks of the zygomatic arch and their influence of the inner facial frame was discussed, and basing the diagnosis on axial CT scans was recommended. The authors stated that the only way to safely expose the entire zygomatic arch was through an extended coronal incision. The surgical approach is described in detail, particularly the location of the frontal branch of the facial nerve in relation to the fascial planes in the temporal region, and the importance of dissecting the coronal flap with the temporoparietal fascia and periosteum over the zygomatic arch. Extensions of the standard approach may be necessary depending on the fracture pattern. Open reduction and internal fixation was mainly done by using miniplates. In secondary reconstructions osteotomies, bone grafting may be necessary to bridge bone gaps and to restore correct orbital volume.

Study Design

An observational case series.

Sample Size

A total of 317 zygomatic arches exposed by coronal incisions for acute trauma during the period 1979–1987, taken from a group of 964 patients treated at their regional trauma centre. Of these, 47 patients had zygomatic arch exposure via a coronal incision for secondary reconstruction of post-traumatic deformities.

Follow-up

No follow-up data was included.

Inclusion/Exclusion Criteria

Not specified.

Intervention or Treatment Received

Primary or secondary reconstruction in midface trauma including access to the zygomatic arch using a coronal flap.

Results

Access to the arch was undertaken before the surgeons had a clear understanding of the anatomy of the temporal region in 15 cases. Out of these, nine patients had a temporary facial nerve palsy, of which four were permanent. Following modification of their access, based on better understanding of the anatomy, there were a further 23 cases of temporary frontal branch palsy seen, and only one permanent palsy, which was likely caused by dissection in the wrong anatomical plane. None of the treated secondary deformity cases had a permanent facial nerve deficit.

A classification of the zygomatic arch fractures separate to the body fracture was proposed together with a treatment protocol derived from this descriptive classification system. For orbitozygomatic fractures, it was suggested that isolated arch fractures and minimally displaced body fractures can be managed with standard techniques. Minimally displaced arch fractures where adequate arch projection is maintained can be managed through local incisions. Where there is a loss of antero-posterior arch projection, a coronal flap was recommended.

With midfacial fractures the arch projection on the fractured side can be compared to the unaffected side, but in bilateral fractures the authors advised to be aware of changes in projection and to compare the shape to normal facial images. In secondary deformity cases, arch projection was most commonly the source of error and full exposure with a coronal flap to allow osteotomy and repositioning was recommended.

Study Limitations

Although the article was clearly a milestone in the field of midface reconstruction, the study lacked objective data to validate the proposed treatment protocols. There was no clear research question, and inclusion or exclusion criteria were not defined. The authors opinion was not supported by any quantifiable measurement or follow-up results, and there was no control group.

Relevant Studies

Since the article is published in 1989, there has been a great deal more literature published in the field of complex midfacial fractures, and standard treatment concepts have been refined. In this section the following topics are discussed: recommendation for imaging, classification, surgical approaches, osteosynthesis, and the use of bone grafts in midfacial fractures.

Imaging in Complex Midfacial Fractures

Ongoing technological advances in computed tomography (CT) with the possibility of three-dimensional (3D) reconstruction have made this the standard for assessing midfacial fractures.[1,2] The CT dataset can then also be used for preoperative surgical planning and computer-assisted surgery (CAS). Contemporary preoperative planning follows the principles that Gruss et al. promoted in reconstructing the outer frame of the midface first, respecting the vertical, transverse and sagittal buttresses. The nonaffected parts of the midface can be mirrored or standard models used to aid the virtual reconstruction.[3]

Reconstruction in complex midfacial fractures can also now be aided by using patient-specific plates and implants that are based on initial CT imaging.[4] Besides using computer-assisted surgery, navigation and patient-specific implants, intraoperative imaging is becoming increasingly important in trying to obtain anatomically correct reconstructions.[5–7]

Classification

In routine clinical practice, fracture classification is typically based on the involved bony structures and their degree of displacement. There are sophisticated classification systems available that allow for an individual fracture mapping in the midface regarding severity, fragmentation, displacement of the fragment, or bone defect, but in the midface, they do not offer a great deal to the clinical decision-making process and are therefore not used.[8–10]

Surgical Approaches

In contrast to the proposed surgical approach to the zygomatic arch by using the coronal incision, there is good evidence for using minimally-invasive approaches to avoid the time-consuming coronal access, which leaves a long scar on the scalp and has the risk of permanent facial nerve weakness. Before using a coronal approach, the combination of an upper eyelid incision with an intraoral approach, with or without a lower eyelid incision, should be discussed.[11] In addition, we would now recommend a retroseptal, transconjunctival approach if access to the orbital rim and inner walls is required.[12] Coronal flap access is generally reserved for more comminuted fractures where there are inadequate reference points anteriorly to enable accurate 3D repositioning of the zygomatic complex and stable fixation.

When a coronal flap is indicated, complete stripping of the insertion of masseter is generally not necessary, and excessive soft tissue stripping (particularly without adequate resuspension during wound closure) can lead to soft tissue sagging, and may increase the risk of bone resorption due to devascularisation.

Osteosynthesis

Since the introduction of stable osteosynthesis in facial trauma, miniplates have become the standard for enabling 3D stability.[13] Resorbable plate fixation has not yet gained widespread acceptance for the treatment of complex midfacial fractures.[14]

Bone Grafts

Historically, bone grafting was frequently used for reconstruction of the orbit and less frequently the lower midface.[15] The indication of bone grafting in primary midfacial reconstruction is reducing markedly with the development of stable titanium osteosynthesis and particularly patient-specific implants to reconstruct defects and contour deformities.[16,17]

REFERENCES

1. Saigal K, Winokur RS, Finden S, et al., Use of three-dimensional computerized tomography reconstruction in complex facial trauma. Facial Plast Surg. 2005; 21: 214–20.
2. Marinaro J, Crandall CS, Doezema D. Computed tomography of the head as a screening examination for facial fractures. Am J Emerg Med. 2007; 25: 616–9.
3. Schramm A, Suarez-Cunqueiro MM, Rücker M, et al. Computer-assisted therapy in orbital and mid-facial reconstructions. Int J Med Robot. 2009; 5: 111–24.
4. Gander T, Essig H, Metzler P, et al. Patient specific implants (PSI) in reconstruction of orbital floor and wall fractures. J Craniomaxillofac Surg. 2015; 43: 126–30.
5. Blumer M, Gander T, Gujer AK, et al. Influence of mirrored computed tomograms on decision-making for revising surgically treated orbital floor fractures. J Oral Maxillofac Surg. 2015; 73: 1982 e1–e9.
6. Gander T, Blumer M, Rostetter C, et al. Intraoperative 3-dimensional cone beam computed tomographic imaging during reconstruction of the zygoma and orbit. Oral Surg Oral Med Oral Pathol Oral Radiol. 2018; 126: 192–7.
7. Pohlenz P, Blake F, Blessmann M, et al. Intraoperative cone-beam computed tomography in oral and maxillofacial surgery using a C-arm prototype: first clinical experiences after treatment of zygomaticomaxillary complex fractures. J Oral Maxillofac Surg. 2009; 67 515–21.
8. Kunz C, Audigé L, Cornelius CP, et al. The comprehensive AOCMF classification system: midface fractures – level 2 tutorial. Craniomaxillofac Trauma Reconstr. 2014; 7: S059–S067.
9. Cornelius CP, Audigé L, Kunz C, et al. The comprehensive AOCMF classification system: midface fractures – level 3 tutorial. Craniomaxillofac Trauma Reconstr. 2014; 7: S068–S091.
10. Kunz C., , Audigé L, Cornelius C-P, et al. The comprehensive AOCMF classification system: orbital fractures – level 3 tutorial. Craniomaxillofac Trauma Reconstr. 2014; 7: S092–S102.
11. Philip JN, Campbell DF. The Edinburgh modification of the minimal access zygomatic osteotomy, used for the correction of zygomatic orbital hypoplasia. Int J Oral Maxillofac Surg. 2017; 46: 1102–5.

12. Gander T, Rostetter C, Blumer M, et al. Use of a monopolar microneedle device in a transconjunctival, retroseptal approach. J Craniomaxillofac Surg. 2017; 45: 1934–7.

13. Wiltfang J. Osteosynthesis systems in mouth, jaw and facial surgery. HNO. 2002; 50: 800–11.

14. Hoffmann J, Troitzsch D, Gülicher D, Adam C, Reinert S. Significance of biodegradable implants in case of midfacial fractures. Biomed Tech (Berl). 2002; 47: 496–9.

15. Manson PN, Crawley WA, Yaremchuk MJ, et al. Midface fractures: advantages of immediate extended open reduction and bone grafting. Plast Reconstr Surg. 1985; 76: 1–12.

16. Parthasarathy J. 3D modeling, custom implants and its future perspectives in craniofacial surgery. Annals of maxillofacial surgery. 2014; 4: 9–18.

17. Guevara-Rojas G, Figl M, Schicho K, et al. Patient-specific polyetheretherketone facial implants in a computer-aided planning workflow. J Oral Maxillofac Surg. 2014; 72: 1801–12.

CHAPTER 48

Computer-Assisted Secondary Reconstruction of Unilateral Post-Traumatic Orbital Deformity

Gellrich NC, Schramm A, Hammer B, et al.
Plast Reconstr Surg. 2002; 110: 1417–29.

Reviewed by Ruud Schreurs and Leander Dubois

Research Question/Objective

The authors have pioneered the field of computer-assisted surgery (CAS) and used preoperative planning, intraoperative navigation, and postoperative evaluation for secondary unilateral orbital reconstructions. Apart from evaluating the use of intraoperative navigation, the objective of the study was to measure two-dimensional and three-dimensional changes of the affected orbit and compare these measures to the unaffected orbit.

Study Design

The study design was a retrospective two centre consecutive cohort study. Surgery for all patients was preplanned using a modified software tool. Intraoperative navigation was used during surgery. A noninvasive registration method, using a dental occlusal splint mounted with four markers, was utilised to correlate the virtual planning to the patient's intraoperative position. No control group was used.

Sample Size

A total of 18 patients who required secondary correction of unilateral post-traumatic orbital deformity were included. The age of the patients ranged from 15 to 61 years; three were female and 15 were male; 12 patients had fractured the left side and six had right-sided injuries.

Follow-up

Radiological follow-up consisted of postoperative computed tomography (CT) scans for all patients. Preoperative radiological measurements were repeated on the postoperative CT scans, to assess volumetric changes and changes in globe projection on the affected side and assess similarity to the unaffected side. No clinical follow-up was described, apart from clinical outcomes achieved in one operation for all patients.

Inclusion/Exclusion Criteria

Patients who underwent secondary reconstruction due to unilateral post-traumatic orbital deformity.

Intervention or Treatment Received

Orbital reconstruction was performed with autologous bone by augmenting one (n = 1), two(n = 7), three (n = 8) or all four (n = 2) walls. In 15 of 18 patients (83%), the zygomaticomaxillary complex (ZMC) was also (re-)osteotomised.

Results

The orbital volume preoperatively was 26.12 cm³ ± 2.85 cm³ (unaffected) and 30.74 cm³ ± 3.57 cm³ (affected). After reconstruction, the mean volume decrease was 4.0 cm³ ± 1.9 cm³, resulting in a mean affected volume of 26.73 cm³ ± 3.39 cm³. The CT-based globe projection preoperatively was 50.76 mm ± 3.20 mm (unaffected) and 48.27 mm ± 4.67 mm (affected). The reconstructed side changed to 54.15 mm ± 3.87 mm, an increase of 5.88 mm ± 2.98 mm. The corrected preoperative Hertel index was 13.92 mm ± 2.70 mm (affected) and 15.78 mm ± 2.11 mm (unaffected); postoperatively the Hertel index changed to 17.29 mm ± 2.96 mm (affected) and 15.96 mm ± 2.05 mm (unaffected).

The decrease in difference in the affected and unaffected sides was significant for both orbital volume, globe projection and CT-based Hertel changes (Student t-test; $p < 0.05$).

The authors stated that the advances in imaging techniques and associated technologies had improved the preoperative planning and surgery. The extra time required for both planning and navigation was 1.5 hour on average. A good clinical outcome was achieved in all patients.

Study Limitations

As the authors did not use a control group with traditional orbital reconstruction and/or did not superimpose the planned contours with the results they achieved, it was not possible to really evaluate the benefit of CAS.

The key results of this study are based on the volume changes after orbital reconstruction with the help of CAS. Unfortunately, the method for measuring the orbital volume is not validated. The differences in the preoperative and postoperative volume in the unaffected side reinforced this inaccuracy.

Another criticism is that the follow-up and the timing of the measurements were not described. Swelling can have a considerable impact on soft tissue volume and the globe projection, which makes the results difficult to interpret. Other fundamental clinical information is lacking, such as amount of diplopia and other clinical sequelae.

Relevant Studies

This study contributed to the beginnings of computer-assisted surgery in oral and maxillofacial surgery. Many larger cohort studies on intraoperative navigation have been performed since, with emphasis of its use in orbital reconstruction. Yu et al. described several indications for intraoperative navigation in a cohort study of 104 patients (ZMC fractures, TMJ ankyloses, fibrous dysplasia, mandibular angle hypertrophia, jaw tumours and foreign bodies).[1] They found a mean error between planning and surgical result of 1.46 ± 0.24 mm and concluded navigation to be a useful supplement.

A matched-control study was performed by Cai et al. to assess the use of intraoperative navigation in orbital reconstruction in 58 patients (29 with navigation, 29 without).[2] Follow-up was performed at 1, 3, 6, and 12 months, where diplopia, hypoesthesia, opthalmoplegia, hypoglobus, and complications were assessed. Patients were found to have a significantly reduced diplopia rate if navigation was used, at 1 month (24% vs. 59%, $p = 0.031$), 3 months (14% vs. 55%, $p = 0.031$), and 12 months (2% vs. 10%, $p = 0.039$) follow-up. No significant differences were found in the other parameters. Implant position was assessed with distance measurements to the mirrored orbit, which was significantly improved in the navigation group ($p = 0.001$).

Bly et al. described 113 consecutive cases, 56 with CAS and 57 without. 90 cases were analysed (45 vs. 45).[3] Diplopia improvement was higher in the navigation group ($p = 0.003$), with an even larger effect in complex fractures ($p < 0.001$). The need for revision surgery was significantly reduced in the navigation group (4% vs. 20%, $p = 0.03$).

The effect of navigation on implant position and restored volume of the orbit using individually bent titanium mesh was radiologically assessed by Essig et al.[4] Navigation was used in 60 patients, compared to 34 historical controls without navigation. Orbital volume was significantly reduced in the navigation group (27.7 ± 3.4 ml to 25.7 ± 3.0 ml, $p < 0.05$), but not in the conventional group (25.6 ± 3.3 ml to 25.3 ± 3.3ml). However, no significant volume differences seemed to be present between the unaffected orbit and the affected orbit in the conventional group.

Zavaterro et al. investigated diplopia severity (0–3 scale), clinical preoperative and postoperative globe position (normal/abnormal), need for revision surgery, complications, operative time, and orbital volume preoperative and postoperative in a study comparing orbital reconstruction with navigation (n = 30) and without navigation (n = 25).[5] A significant volume reduction was achieved in the navigation group, but not in the conventional group. The scatter plot comparing unaffected and reconstructed volume seems to indicate better performance on an individual level in the navigation group. The secondary operation rate was 20% in the conventional group and 0% in the navigation group.

A prospective, multicentre study was performed by Zimmerer et al.[6] A total of 195 patients were included and were divided in two groups: a group using individualised implants (n = 95, ranging from free-hand bending to PSI) and a group using preformed implants (n = 100). In the individualised group, navigation was used in 55.8% of cases, in the conventional group in 18.0%. The primary aim was to compare the precision of the reconstruction in terms of volume; secondary clinical outcome parameters included globe position, visual acuity, motility, and diplopia. The individualised group performed better in terms of reconstructed volume compared to the unaffected orbit.

A cadaveric one-on-one comparison of the effects of intraoperative navigation in orbital reconstruction was performed by Dubois et al.[7] The same 19 defects were reconstructed twice: once with the help of navigation and once without navigation. The primary outcome measures were rotation and translation of the acquired implant position compared to the planned position. Intraoperative navigation was demonstrated to lead to better implant positioning and a more predictable reconstruction of the same defect in terms of translation (p = 0.002), roll (p = 0.001) and yaw (p < 0.001).

Two systematic reviews about the use of intraoperative navigation in craniomaxillofacial surgery have been published, both concluding support from the collective published data for the use of intraoperative navigation in craniofacial trauma, and especially orbital reconstruction.[8,9] A general consensus seems to exist that precision of implant positioning is enhanced if intraoperative navigation is used.

In the current study, autologous bone was used for reconstruction of the orbital defect. In 2003, Ellis et al. concluded in a series of 58 patients with unilateral blowout fractures that a more accurate reconstruction could be achieved with titanium mesh implants; other advantages of titanium mesh over autologous bone include easier handling and manipulation.[10] In the period following this publication, the implant material of choice has shifted away from autologous bone.

Currently, laser-sintered patient-specific implants are the most technologically advanced option.[11-13] They are highly compatible with the concepts of preoperative planning and intraoperative navigation, since their optimal position (and in the case of a PSI even the optimal shape) can be determined in the preoperative planning phase.

The accuracy of intraoperative navigation, and its feedback reliability, is greatly dependent on the initial registration accuracy. Dental-worn registration splints with appropriate markers are still in use because of their unique fit and easy reinsertion during surgery. Maxillary bone screws are used as an alternative.[1,5] Several studies have investigated registration methods for oral and maxillofacial surgery and have verified the overall accuracy of 1–1.5 mm, which was qualitatively assessed in the results of this study.[14–16]

REFERENCES

1. Yu H, Shen SG, Wang X, Zhang L, Zhang S. The indication and application of computer-assisted navigation in oral and maxillofacial surgery — Shanghai's experience based on 104 cases. J Cranio-Maxillofac Surg. 2013; 41: 770–4.
2. Cai EZ, Koh YP, Hing ECH, et al. Computer-assisted navigational surgery improves outcomes in orbital reconstructive surgery. J Craniofac Surg. 2012; 23: 1567–73.
3. Bly R, Chang SH, Cudejkova M, Liu JJ, Moe KS. Computer-guided orbital reconstruction to improve outcomes. J Am Med Assoc Facial Plas Surg. 2013; 15: 113–20.
4. Essig H, Dressel L, Rana M, et al. Precision of posttraumatic primary orbital reconstruction using individually bent titanium mesh with and without navigation: a retrospective study. Head Face Med. 2013; 9: 18.
5. Zavattero E, Ramieri G, Roccia F, Gerbino G. Comparison of the outcomes of complex orbital fracture repair with and without a surgical navigation system: a prospective cohort study with historical controls. Plas Recon Surg. 2017; 139: 957–65.
6. Zimmerer R, Ellis III E, Aniceto GS, et al. A prospective multicentre study to compare the precision of posttraumatic internal orbital reconstruction with standard preformed and individualized orbital implants. J Cranio-Maxillofac Surg. 2016; 44: 1485–97.
7. Dubois L, Schreurs R, Jansen J, et al. Predictability in orbital reconstruction: a human cadaver study. Part II: navigation-assisted orbital reconstruction. J Cranio-Maxillofac Surg. 2015; 43: 2042–49.
8. Azarmehr I, Stokbro K, Bell RB, Thygesen T. Surgical navigation: a systematic review of indications, treatments, and outcomes in oral and maxillofacial surgery. J Oral Maxillofac Surg. 2017; 75: 1987–2005.
9. DeLong MR, Gandolfi BM, Barr ML, et al. Intraoperative image-guided navigation in craniofacial surgery: review and grading of the current literature. J Craniofac Surg. 2019; 30: 465–72.
10. Ellis IIIE, Tan Y. Assessment of internal orbital reconstructions for pure blowout fractures: cranial bone grafts versus titanium mesh. J Oral Maxillofac Surg. 2003; 61: 442–53.
11. Stoor P, Suomalainen A, Lindqvist C, et al. Rapid prototyped patient specific implants for reconstruction of orbital wall defects. J Cranio-Maxillofac Surg. 2014; 42: 1644–9.
12. Gander T, Essig H, Metzler P, et al. Patient specific implants (PSI) in reconstruction of orbital floor and wall fractures. J Cranio-Maxillofac Surg. 2015; 43: 126–30.

13. Rana M, Chui CH, Wagner M, et al. Increasing the accuracy of orbital reconstruction with selective laser-melted patient-specific implants combined with intraoperative navigation. J Oral Maxillofac Surg. 2015; 73: 1113–8.

14. Luebbers HT, Messmer P, Obwegeser JA, et al. Comparison of different registration methods for surgical navigation in cranio-maxillofacial surgery. J Cranio-Maxillofac Surg. 2008; 36: 109–16.

15. Essig H, Rana M, Kokemueller H, et al. Referencing of markerless CT data sets with cone beam subvolume including registration markers to ease computer-assisted surgery – a clinical and technical research. Int J Medic Robot Comp Assist Surg. 2013; 9: e39–e45.

16. Venosta D, Sun Y, Matthews F, et al. Evaluation of two dental registration-splint techniques for surgical navigation in cranio-maxillofacial surgery. J Cranio-Maxillofac Surg. 2014; 42: 448–53.

CHAPTER 49

Management of the Medial Canthal Tendon in Nasoethmoid Orbital Fractures: The Importance of the Central Fragment in Classification and Treatment

Markowitz BL, Manson PN, Sargent L, et al.
Plast Reconstr Surg. 1991; 87: 843–53.

Reviewed by Baucke van Minnen

Research Question/Objective

Before publication of this article many papers had already addressed the anatomy of the naso-orbital-ethmoid (NOE) region and the challenges in treatment of fractures in this complex region.[1-3] In other previous studies, restoration of the intercanthal dimensions and the reattachment of the medial canthal tendon was also addressed.[4,5] However, as treatment methods had improved after the introduction of miniplate and screw systems, changes in the diagnostic classification in relation to the treatment were necessary. Before 1991, no publication had defined the injury pattern of the medial orbital rim in relation to the modern operative and fixation techniques available for treatment. The objective of this publication was to classify the fracture pattern of the bony fragment on which the medial canthal tendon inserts (the "central fragment"). This classification relates the severity of the injury to the degree of exposure and fixation necessary for adequate treatment.

Study Design

A consecutive case series at the Maryland Institute of Emergency Medical Service Systems. All patients receiving operative treatment for acute NOE fractures were included.

Sample Size

A total of 234 consecutive patients during the years 1976–1986.

Follow-up

Three months to 3 years.

Inclusion Criteria

Diagnosis of displaced or mobile naso-orbito-ethmoid fracture necessitating operative treatment.

Intervention or Treatment Received

From 1976 to 1984 plate and screw systems were not available, and operative treatment was performed without plate and screw fixation (n = 164). From 1985–1986 surgical management was done with plate and screw fixation if possible (n = 72).

Results

Before 1985, and without CT data, fractures could only be classified as unilateral or bilateral and isolated to the central part of the midface or extended. Analysis of the fracture patterns in patients managed from 1985 refined the classification by identifying the fracture pattern in the central fragment. The central fragment can exist as a single segment with intact attachment of the medial canthal tendon, classified as a Type I injury (Figure 49.1). Type I injuries can be further subdivided into displaced or nondisplaced fractures and unilateral or bilateral fractures. Comminution of the central fragment may occur without involvement of the medial canthal insertion (Type II injury, Figure 49.1). If the fractures of the comminuted central fragment extend into the bone providing the canthal insertion, the fracture is classified as Type III (Figure 49.2). In Type III complete canthal avulsion from the bone may be present.

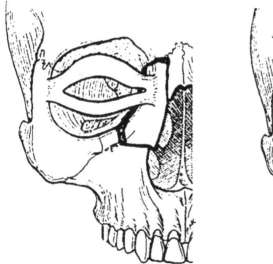 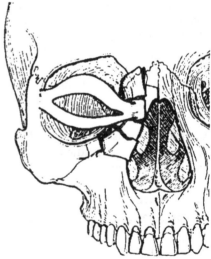

Figure 49.1 (Composed from Figures 3 and 4 from the original article): Type I injury (left). Type II injury (right). In Type II injuries the bone fractures do not extend into the area of canthal insertion.

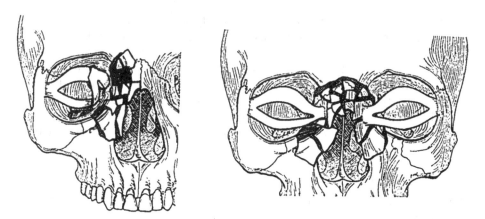

Figure 49.2   Type III injuries. Bone fractures extend into the bone providing canthal insertion (right). Canthal avulsion may be present (left).

The required surgical exposure and type of fixation was described in relation to the fracture pattern. Inferior approaches were performed for unilateral Type I injuries that were non-displaced superiorly. The lower eyelid subciliary skin approach and the maxillary intraoral approach were both used. The authors stated that a combination of superior and inferior approaches is necessary for displaced unilateral Type I injuries, for bilateral Type I injuries, and all comminuted fractures.

Once the fractures were exposed, Type I injuries were stabilised with junctional plate and screw fixation. The number and position of the plates varied with the location of the displacement. In comminuted fractures (Type II and III), a nasoethmoid unit was created by linking the bone segments with inter-fragment wires. As the fracture in Type III injuries extends through the bone providing the canthal insertion, the latter was detached from the bone before reduction. In Type II fractures the canthus was not detached. The reduced nasoethmoid unit was fixed to the frontal bone and orbital rims with plate and screws. Furthermore, both Type II and III injuries were treated with transnasal wiring.

Additional bone grafting to the nasal dorsum of the nose was used in 66% of the bilateral comminuted fractures. Additional treatment of the lacrimal system was and final outcome were not described.

Study Limitations

The authors gave a detailed description of the fracture classification of the central fragment. This classification is helpful in scientific reports and in clinical treatment, as it is well described and reproducible by others. The treatments described by the authors can be defined as an expert opinion. They are clear about the plate fixation of the Type I injuries and the indication for transnasal wiring in Type II and III injuries. It is not clearly described what the indications for additional bone grafting of the nasal dorsum and septum were. The authors stated that successful outcome of NOE fractures is dependent on reduction and stabilisation of the central fragment of the fracture with its medial canthal tendon. Although this statement has been supported by many others in the decades after this report, the authors do not clearly describe their parameters for failure or success in their original article. Unfavourable outcome, including telecanthus, was mentioned in general in the discussion section, but the outcome of their own research population was not clear.

Relevant Studies

Review articles published on the treatment of NOE fractures show that the classification by Markowitz is still widely accepted.[6,7] It is recognised that the meticulous reduction and stabilisation of the canthal ligament or the canthus-bearing bony segment is the key to successful restoration of the pre-trauma facial appearance.[8] For the required surgical exposure, it is still advised to combine a superior exposure by way of a coronal approach with a lower local approach in cases with comminution and displacement. Since publication of this article, the transconjunctival approach with a possible trans-caruncular extension has gained popularity.[9] Nevertheless, skin incisions are still promoted. The usefulness of the different approaches is dependent on the presence of lacerations and the particular area that needs to be reached for fixation.

Fixation of the displaced Type I injuries with miniplates and screws has not been subject to debate since this paper has been published. Markowitz described that canthopexy is always necessary in Type II and Type III injuries. However, possibly as a result of the increased experience with plate and screw systems, more recent reports state that Type II injuries can be treated with plate fixation, as long as the small segments are "plateable."[10,11] The method of medial canthopexy by transnasal wiring is still an accepted procedure. Complementary to transnasal wiring, reattachment of the canthal ligament with aid of a miniplate and a wire (metal or anchored wire system) was described.[12–14] The miniplate is fixated to the nasal or frontal bone and extends posteriorly into the orbit, facilitating the reposition of the posterior limb of the medial canthal ligament.

In conclusion, over 25 years after publication, the Markowitz classification has been proven to be very useful in determining the severity of the fracture and is still the basis for diagnostic classification of NOE fractures. In the original article the proposed treatment strategy cannot be correlated with outcome, and therefore many modifications in approaches, fixation of bone segments and canthopexy have been published since.

REFERENCES

1. Dingman RO, Grabb WC, Oneal RM. Management of injuries of the naso-orbital complex. Arch Surg. 1969; 98: 566–71.
2. Duvall AJ, Banovetz JD. Nasoethmoidal fractures. Otolaryngol Clin North Am. 1976; 9: 507–15.
3. Morgan RF, Manson PN, Shack RB, Hoopes JE. Management of naso-ethmoid-orbital fractures. Am Surg. 1982; 48: 447–50.
4. Converse JM, Smith B. Naso-orbital fractures and traumatic deformities of the medial canthus. Plast Reconstr Surg. 1966; 38: 147–62.
5. Zide BM, McCarthy JG. The medial canthus revisited – An anatomical basis for canthopexy. Ann Plast Surg. 1983; 11: 1–9.
6. Papadopoulos H, Salib NK. Management of naso-orbital-ethmoidal fractures. Oral Maxillofac Surg Clin North Am. 2009; 21: 221–5.
7. Wei JJ, Tang ZL, Liu L, et al. The management of naso-orbital-ethmoid (NOE) fractures. Chin J Traumatol. 2015; 18: 296–301.
8. Parashar A, Sharma RK. Unfavourable outcomes in maxillofacial injuries: how to avoid and manage. Indian J Plast Surg. 2013; 46: 221–34.
9. Al-Moraissi EA, Thaller SR, Ellis E. Subciliary vs. transconjunctival approach for the management of orbital floor and periorbital fractures: a systematic review and meta-analysis. J Craniomaxillofac Surg. 2017; 45: 1647–54.
10. Antonyshyn O. Nasoorbitoethmoidal (NOE) fractures. In Ehrenfeld M, Manson PN, Prein J (Eds.): Principles of Internal Fixation of the Craniomaxillofacial Skeleton. Stuttgart: Thieme, 2012.
11. Booth PW. Naso-ethmoid fractures. In: Hearle F, Champy M (Eds.): Atlas of Craniomaxillofacial Osteosynthesis. Stuttgart: Thieme, 2009.
12. Hammer B. Orbital Fractures – diagnosis, Operative Treatment, Secondary Corrections, 1st ed. Cambridge: Hogrefe & Huber, 1995.
13. Wittkampf AR, Mourits MP. A simple method for medial canthal reconstruction. Int J Oral Maxillofac Surg. 2001; 30: 342–3.
14. Engelstad ME, Bastodkar P, Markiewicz MR. Medial canthopexy using transcaruncular barb and miniplate: technique and cadaver study. Int J Oral Maxillofac Surg. 2012; 41: 1176–85.

CHAPTER 50

Twenty-Six-Year Experience Treating Frontal Sinus Fractures: A Novel Algorithm Based on Anatomical Fracture Pattern and Failure of Conventional Techniques

Rodriguez ED, Stanwix MG, Nam AJ, et al.
Plast Reconstr Surg. 2008; 122: 1850–66.

Reviewed by Eric J Dierks

Research Question/Objective

Although the international literature is replete with case reports and small series of frontal sinus fractures, few studies have undergone rigorous statistical analysis. The myriad of proposed treatment protocols therefore tend to be the product of local tradition and personal preference rather than evidence-based. This study aimed to produce a validated treatment algorithm based on the considerable experience of the R. Adams Cowley Shock Trauma Centre in Baltimore, Maryland, USA of frontal sinus fractures.

Study Design

This retrospective, single centre review identified frontal sinus fracture patients from 1979 to 2005. Fractures were categorised by location, displacement, comminution, and naso-frontal outflow tract (NFOT) injury as defined by the presence of one or more of the following three criteria.[1] outflow tract/ductal "obstruction",[2] frontal sinus floor fracture,[3] fracture of the medial aspect of the anterior table.

Demographic data, treatment modalities, and complications were compiled. Acute "major" complications were defined as those occurring within six months that required surgery, and complications that did not require surgery were termed "minor." The patients were divided by site of fracture: nondisplaced anterior wall (21.6%), displaced anterior wall (16.7%), nondisplaced posterior wall (3.6%), displaced posterior wall (3.3%), nondisplaced anterior and posterior table (16.5%), and displaced anterior and posterior table (38.4%). Patients within each of these patient groups were further divided into treatment modality utilised, complications, and which of the three above-noted criteria of NFOT injury were met.

Three services treat frontal sinus fractures at this trauma centre: plastic surgery, oral and maxillofacial surgery, and otolaryngology. The treating service for each patient was not specified.

Inclusion/Exclusion Criteria

Inclusion criteria were all patients with frontal sinus fractures admitted to the R. Adams Cowley Shock Trauma Centre in Baltimore, Maryland, USA from 1979 to 2005.

Exclusion criteria were those patients whose clinical or radiographic records were incomplete or if they had undergone decompressive craniectomy without subsequent frontal sinus surgery. Patients who died within 48 hours without treatment were also excluded.

Sample Size

Of a total of 1097 frontal sinus fracture patients identified, 153 were excluded due to insufficient data and 87 were excluded due to death within 48 hours without treatment, resulting in a robust cohort size of 857. Of this group, 504 patients (58.8%) underwent surgery and the remainder were managed by observation.

Follow-up

Patient follow-up averaged 2.8 months, with a range of 0–66 months. The average length of convalescence prior to return to work or function was 114 days.

Intervention or Treatment Received

The CT scans of all patients were reviewed and the patients were categorised with specific attention to the presence/absence of NFOT injury. Although not specified, it is presumed that the CT scans were reviewed retrospectively by the authors. Treatment modalities included observation, reconstruction with outflow tract and mucosal preservation, obliteration, osteoneogenesis, and cranialisation.

Results

Motor vehicle collision was the most common injury mechanism (42%) with an additional 10% of cases due to motorcycle collision. A majority of patients (70.7%) had NFOT injury and 67% had a diagnosis of obstruction. Of the 504 patients that underwent surgery, 10.4% experienced a complication as compared to a 3.1% complication rate among the 353 patients that were observed. In both

Table 50.1   Associated injuries in frontal sinus fractures with and without nasofrontal outflow tract injury

Injury	Without NFOT Injury (%)	With NFOT Injury (%)
Brain	31	76
Cervical spine	7	14
Upper extremity fracture	15	25
Lower extremity fracture	13	23
Pneumothorax	12	24
Abdominal	7	13
Orbital roof	13	40
Orbital wall	7	13
Orbital floor	2	7
NOE	12	31
Zygoma	8	18
Le Fort	2	17
Mandible	3	5

NOE, nasoorbitoethmoid complex; NFOT, nasofrontal outflow tract.

groups, all complications except for one occurred among patients with NFOT injury. That single complication patient without NFOT injury had undergone NFOT stenting. The authors opine that the complication might have not happened had the patient been observed and not stented.

Central to this study's focus on NFOT injury is Table 50.1, "Associated Injuries," which were listed both with and without NFOT injury. Fractures of adjacent facial bones were subdivided in Table 50.1, and NFOT injury injured patients were found to have three times more concomitant facial fractures than those without. The most highly associated injury was brain. An associated (unspecified) brain injury was present among 76% of frontal sinus fracture patients with NFOT injury and 31% without. Naso-orbital-ethmoid (NOE) fractures were also associated with frontal sinus fractures; 31% with NFOT injury and 12% without.

Of the surgical options, cranialisation was found to be the most common, obliteration was second, and reconstruction third. The most common material used for obliteration was bone (34% of obliterations).

Of the 504 patients that underwent surgery, 94% had nasofrontal tract injury by at least one criterion, with "obstruction" being observed in 77%. Major complications were seen among 61 patients (7.1%) and only 1 patient in this group did not have NFOT injury. The 41 patients who underwent fat obliteration experienced a 22% complication rate, whereas only 6% of those obliterated with materials other than fat experienced a complication. Obliteration with vascularised pericranium, popularised in 1994 by Thaller and Donald[1] and commonly used today, was not specifically mentioned.

The authors employed the receiver operating characteristic under the curve statistical analysis to validate their management algorithm. Their value of 0.8621 indicates a diagnostic accuracy of over 86%, which is regarded as statistically significant.

Study Limitations

This study shares the limitations that are inherent in any long-term retrospective review. The average follow-up is short, as is common among other studies of maxillofacial trauma. The patients were not treated on a protocol, and the backgrounds, priorities, and goals of the various treating surgeons probably differed and may well have evolved over the long duration of this study. Multiple faculty surgeons within several surgical disciplines managed the patients enrolled in this study. The progress of technology marched onward during the 26-year span of this study, as it has since the study's completion. The quality of computed tomography (CT) imaging of the frontal sinus and nasofrontal outflow region has improved dramatically since the beginning of this study in 1979, arousing some question regarding the actual radiographic presence or absence of NFOT injury. Xie et al. stated in their 30-year retrospective review of 150 frontal fracture patients that "the function of the frontal sinus is notoriously difficult to predict from radiographic patterns"[2] which challenges the Rodriguez group's assessment of NFOT injury based on CT scan review.

The most notable relevant technological surgical advancement since 1979 has been the development of endoscopic surgery of the paranasal sinuses. Although routine endoscopic access to the area of the nasofrontal duct and frontal recess areas was not common during the early part of this study, this technology and its related skill set have evolved considerably during the latter part of this study's duration. If any endoscopic approaches were utilised either acutely or secondarily, this was not noted. There is no mention of how many patients underwent secondary endoscopic sinus surgery for nasofrontal outflow obstruction. This is understandable given the short length of patient follow-up in this and other similar studies. Therefore, the focus on NFOT injury and obstruction as read on CT scans may be inappropriate in the age of advanced nasal endoscopic surgical techniques that definitively manage outflow obstruction.

Relevant Studies

In 1970, Mark May et al. reviewed 21 frontal sinus fracture patients and noted nasofrontal duct injury among 20 of his 21 patients.[3] He added "integrity of the nasofrontal duct" to the list of indications for surgery in frontal sinus fractures. Paul Donald's 1979 monograph utilised a cat model to demonstrate the tenacity of the frontal sinus mucosa.[4] Donald pointed out that "the mucosa dips into the small pits that pockmark the bone," referring to the pits of the diploic veins of

Breschet, as was previously described by Mosher and Judd.[5] These microscopic remnants of sinus mucosa were the source of mucosal regrowth from residual frontal sinus mucosa that were not removed by curettage alone. Donald advocated actual bone removal in this classic paper in which he admonished "surgical colleagues in related disciplines," i.e. neurosurgeons, who only curetted out the mucosa. The concept of leaving a "safe sinus" following frontal sinus trauma emanated from this concept and has guided surgeons of all related disciplines since.

Strong's 2009 publication on the endoscopic reduction of anterior table frontal sinus fractures is one of several that have taken the topic of acute management of frontal sinus fractures into the endoscopic era.[6] Draf has described the delayed endoscopic management of frontal sinus fractures that widely and permanently opens frontal sinus drainage.[7] The 2007 retrospective series of 116 frontal sinus fractures by Bell et al. showed a slightly higher overall complication rate of 16% among operated patients, with a 7.8% rate of complications among those surgical cases involving preservation of the frontal sinus.[8]

Kim et al. reported an eyelid incision approach that allows blunt internal elevation of depressed anterior table elements with endoscopic confirmation of reduction, which in the absence of overlying lacerations, avoids a bicoronal incision.[9] A variation on this theme is offered by Mavili, utilising a percutaneous screw for fragment reduction.[10] Guy and Brissett's review provides an excellent overview of this topic.[11] Of interest to surgeons of any discipline involved in frontal sinus trauma is the 2009 paper by Manson et al. describing their classification of frontobasal skull fractures, which can accompany frontal sinus fractures.[12]

REFERENCES

1. Thaller SR, Donald P. The use of pericranial flaps in frontal sinus fractures. Ann Plast Surg. 1994; 32: 284–7.
2. Xie C, Mehendale N, Barrett D, et al. 30-year retrospective review of frontal sinus fractures: the Charity Hospital experience. J Cranio Maxillofac Trauma. 2000; 6: 7–14.
3. May M, Ogura JH, Schramm V. Nasofrontal duct in frontal sinus fractures. Arch Otolaryngol. 1970; 92: 534–8.
4. Donald PJ. The tenacity of the frontal sinus mucosa. Otolaryngol Head Neck Surg. 1979; 87: 557–66.
5. Mosher HP, Judd DK. An analysis of seven cases of osteomyelitis if the frontal bone complicating frontal sinusitis. Laryngoscope. 1933; 43: 153–212.
6. Strong EB. Endoscopic repair of anterior table frontal sinus fractures. Facial Plast Surg. 2009; 25: 43–8.
7. Draf W. Endonasal micro-endoscopic frontal sinus surgery: the Fulda concept. Op Tech Otolaryngol Head Neck Surg. 1991; 2: 234–40.

8. Bell RB, Dierks EJ, Brar P, Potter JK, Potter BE. A protocol for the management of frontal sinus fractures emphasizing sinus preservation. J Oral Maxillofac Surg. 2007; 65: 825–39.

9. Kim K, Kim E, Hwang J, et al. Transcutaneous transfrontal approach through a small peri-eyebrow incision for the reduction of closed anterior table frontal sinus fractures. J Plast Recon Aesthet Surg. 2010; 63: 763–8.

10. Mavili ME, Canter HI. Closed treatment of frontal sinus fracture with percutaneous screw reduction. J Craniofac Surg. 2007; 18: 415–9.

11. Guy WM, Brissett AE. Contemporary management of traumatic fractures of the frontal sinus. Otolaryngol Clin North Am. 2013; 46: 733–48.

12. Manson PN, Stanwix MG, Yaremchuk MJ, et al. Frontobasal fractures: anatomical classification and clinical significance. Plast Recon Surg. 2009; 124: 2096–106.

Index

Printed in the United States
by Baker & Taylor Publisher Services